Anti-D Explained

Dr Sara Wickham

Anti-D Explained
Published 2021 by Birthmoon Creations
Avebury, Wiltshire
© 2021 Sara Wickham
www.sarawickham.com

Sara Wickham has asserted her moral right to be named as the author of this work in accordance with the Copyright, Designs and Patents Act of 1988.

ISBN: 978-1999806453
Also available as an e-book

This book offers general information for interest only and does not constitute or replace individualised professional midwifery or medical care and advice. Whilst every effort has been made to ensure the accuracy and currency of the information herein, the author accepts no liability or responsibility for any loss or damage caused, or thought to be caused, by making decisions based upon the information in this book and recommends that you use it in conjunction with other trusted sources of information.

About the Author

Dr Sara Wickham PhD, MA, PGCert, BA(Hons) is an author, speaker and researcher who works independently; speaking, writing, teaching online courses and workshops, consulting and creating resources for health professionals, birth workers, writers and others.

Sara's career has been varied; she has lived and worked in the UK, the USA and New Zealand, edited three professional journals and lectured in more than twenty-five countries.

You can find and follow Sara online at her website, www.sarawickham.com, where she writes a blog and offers a free monthly newsletter sharing birth-related information.

Sara is also on Instagram as @DrSaraWickham.

Also by Sara Wickham

Acknowledgements

This book is for the women and families whose questions and desire for better information than is provided in standard information leaflets has led me on a fascinating career and taken me around the world to share my work and research. It's also for a dear midwife friend, Kim Woodard Osterholzer, who lovingly nagged me to write it for nearly a decade!

I want to thank the many midwives, doctors, scientists and others who have supported me on these journeys. I want to begin by crediting those I acknowledged in my first (2001) book in which I share my initial research: Jon Burke, Huguette Comerasamy, Lorna Davies, Robbie Davis-Floyd, Judy Edmunds, Valerie El Halta, Anne Gridley, Mark Horridge, Martin Pooley, Mary Stewart, Jan Tritten and Naoli Vinaver.

I also want to thank those who have supported and helped my ongoing journey of researching and writing about this area, including those who have helped midwife this book: Julie Frohlich, Nadine Edwards, Kirsten Small, Penny Champion, Emma Mills, Gill Boden, Lucyann Ashdown, Jude Davis, Mavis Kirkham, Michel Odent and Ina May Gaskin.

And by no means least, neither this book, nor the first, nor all those in between would have happened without the love and support of my family, most especially my mum and dad (who gave me the use of their dining room table and made me endless meals and cups of tea while I wrote my first book on this topic), Chris, Deb, Rich, and a number of beloved cats, who (while some are more helpful than others) provide an important kind of companionship to writers.

Contents

Foreword

Sara Wickham has found an original way to raise judicious yet unusual questions. Thanks to her exceptional capacity for lateral thinking she has developed the art of 'hitting the nail on the head.'

Try explaining to an intelligent outsider that, for about 50 years, millions of RhD negative women have been routinely injected with an Anti-D immunoglobulin when they gave birth or when they had a miscarriage. Explain also that in fact such an injection was not useful for 90% of these women. The intelligent outsider will probably ask what research has been done to detect the 10% who really need the Anti-D.

Not only does Sara Wickham raise the right question, but she is also in a position to interpret the lack of interest for such an issue in medical circles. She knows how comfortable the obstetricians are with the concept of routine.

Before the recent development of evidence based medicine, it was commonplace to justify routine ultrasound scans and routine electronic fetal monitoring. It is still usual today, in certain obstetrical departments, to practise routine episiotomies, routine artificial ruptures of membranes, etc…

There is a fundamental incompatibility, on the other hand between the art of midwifery and strict protocols which include the word routine. The practice of authentic midwifery presumes that every mother and every baby is a particular case. The current gap between the obstetrical attitude and the midwifery attitude is thoroughly illustrated by the questions they inspire.

The collateral questions raised by Sara are as unusual as the main one: What are the potential risks of infections by known or undiscovered pathogens? Can an ABO-incompatibility reduce the risks of Rh isoimmunisation? Does birth in physiological conditions reduce the risks of Rh isoimmunisation?

The genuine pioneers are those who raise the right questions at the right time.

I wrote this as an introduction to Sara's research on anti-D twenty years ago. My words are still just as relevant today.

Michel Odent
Primal Health Research Centre. London, 2021.

Introduction

For quite a few years now, practitioners of modern medicine (and many other fields) have been embracing an approach which is known as evidence-informed practice. In simple terms, this means we use the results of well-designed research studies to inform the treatments and interventions offered to those seeking care. Research evidence isn't the only form of knowledge that we use to inform practice (if we are health care professionals) or our own decisions about our own health care, and that's why I prefer the term 'evidence-informed' to 'evidence-based'. It's also the case that, even if evidence shows that one or other thing is beneficial at a population level, it's still up to the individual to decide whether it's right for them. But the general idea is that, where possible, we should look to research and science to see if things work, rather than relying mainly on experience.

Many midwives, doctors and other birth attendants have been working hard to get this approach embedded into maternity care. There was a real need for this. That's because a lot of what is offered in modern maternity care was based on tradition and what people *thought* might help, rather than on the results of robust studies showing that something is effective. So, when many of the interventions that had become a standard part of care during pregnancy and childbirth – such as artificial rupture of the membranes (breaking the waters), episiotomy (a cut to help the baby be born) and cardiotocography (also known as CTG or continuous electronic fetal heart rate monitoring) – have been carefully researched, we haven't always found good evidence that they are valuable on a routine basis.

In fact, when held up to close scrutiny, it turns out that many of the interventions introduced into 'normal' childbirth are futile, and often potentially harmful, when used on a routine basis. They can be helpful on occasion, but not for everyone, or when used all the time. This does not mean that the interventions have been removed from practice. Sadly, as I have discussed in previous books (Wickham 2018a), some interventions are still routinely offered in many areas because of fear of litigation and 'just in case,' despite a lack of evidence to support their helpfulness. But we can see that healthy women and their babies may have better outcomes if we respect physiology and allow their journeys of pregnancy and childbirth to unfold without routine intervention.

Please allow me to clarify a few things about that statement though. First, the key word in what I have written above is 'routine.' Routine intervention is the problem. To question the routine application of intervention is not to question any use of intervention; far from it. Caesarean sections are a great example of an intervention that can be lifesaving in a small number of situations. But they are grossly overused, especially in high-income countries and in settings where health care providers and systems of care are paid depending on outcomes or results. As caesareans carry many negative consequences, overuse does more harm than good. The same is true of the use of intravenous oxytocin to induce or augment labour. It can sometimes be helpful to do this, but overuse is rife and causes many problems. So it is generally best to use caesareans, drugs to induce or speed up labour and other interventions judiciously; in other words, only when there is a really good reason to do so.

The second key point that I need to clarify relates to something we call agency; the ability of an individual person to make their own decisions. As I have already mentioned, the decision to have any intervention is made by the person who is being offered the intervention. The role of the health care provider is to offer good information – which should include a sound and fair appraisal of the available evidence – on which a person can base their decision. Whatever the evidence says, it's still up to the person themselves to decide whether something is right for them. But there is, again, a gap between the theory and the reality in some parts of the world. This should apply to all medical care, not just in maternity, but it doesn't always happen. What's important here is to know that this is what should happen, and it's entrenched in many countries' laws and articles of human rights. That doesn't always mean that one can insist on having an intervention if a medical provider doesn't think it's in your best interest. It does mean that any adult with mental capacity can decline care, screening or treatment that they don't want.

I mention these issues before even introducing the topic of this book because they are pivotal to its discussion. I also want to begin this book, as I have done in many of my others, by giving you a bit of information about my own viewpoint and story. That's because I think it's important that you know the source of any information you are reading, so that you can judge its value. I hope you will judge other sources of information too. If everybody was honest about their qualifications, knowledge, beliefs and the approach they take to the evidence that they share, it might be easier to navigate the mass of information – and misinformation – available to us these days.

In 1997, just a few years after I first qualified as a midwife in the UK, I was undertaking a Master's and needed to pick a topic for my dissertation. One of my ideas was to look at the evidence for giving routine Anti-D by injection after the birth of a baby. Anti-D is a medicine made from blood which is offered to certain women in the hope of preventing their future babies from developing a condition known as rhesus disease, or haemolytic disease of the fetus and newborn (HDFN). The women who are offered Anti-D are those who have rhesus negative blood and who have given birth to a baby with rhesus positive blood. I'll explain exactly what all of those terms mean in chapter one.

I had good reason to be considering this matter at that time. Over the previous year or two, a couple of the women who I had cared for as an independent midwife – and who knew that they had rhesus negative blood – had asked me during pregnancy whether Anti-D (or Rhogam®, as it is known in the USA and some other countries) was truly necessary for them. I had to tell them that I didn't know the answer to this question. I realised that I had very little to offer these women beyond the standard information contained in the leaflets made by the companies that produced this particular medicine. These were very basic, and (at least at the time) merely gave an explanation of what Anti-D was, why it was deemed necessary and when it would be given. There was little expectation of anyone questioning this intervention, and the leaflets were written as if compliance was a given.

As I chatted with fellow students and pondered Anti-D as a possible research topic, I realised something else. Anti-D was the only pregnancy and birth-related intervention I could think of which I hadn't previously heard anyone question, challenge or decline. That was surprising to me. Along with many midwives educated in that era, I had learned that there were different ideologies and approaches within the field of childbirth. There still are. Some people take a very medical approach, thinking that lots of intervention and monitoring the physical aspects of birth is best. Some go to the other end of the spectrum and try to avoid every intervention possible. There are many shades of variation in between.

My colleagues and I understood the different approaches. We were living through the beginning of the era of evidence-informed midwifery. We were looking at evidence *and* looking after women. We understood that interventions had downsides as well as benefits. We were used to considering both (or more) sides of the picture. But, until those two women asked me about Anti-D, I hadn't ever heard anyone question that particular intervention. I had spent four years undertaking a direct-entry midwifery degree in the city that was the home of evidence-based medicine. I was amongst a group of lecturers and fellow midwifery students committed to exploring the evidence and the different viewpoints on every topic. So the fact that no-one had really questioned this intervention was a surprising realisation. Why was this intervention so accepted? And, if birth works better for the vast majority of the time without routine intervention, then what made Anti-D the exception to the rule? These were intriguing questions, and one of the reasons this topic interested me was that I felt a little like I was setting out on the trail of a mystery.

Given that you've read the title of this book, there are no prizes for guessing that I decided to research Anti-D. Initially, it took me deep into the stacks of medical libraries in Oxford and London. This was the era of Web 1.0, when not every home had a computer and journals were still printed on paper. I was digging into research that was already nearly thirty years old, and the journals were dusty and yellow. I soon realised that I needed a better understanding of haematology, and of the tests and processes used in this area. So I also spent some time in hospital laboratories with some very patient haematologists and scientific officers.

I'll tell you more about my research and what I learned about Anti-D throughout this book of course. But the more personal side of that story is that what I found in my research was deemed interesting enough at the time that I was asked to write a book about it. Published by Books for Midwives Press (which later became part of the Elsevier family), *Anti-D in Midwifery: Panacea or Paradox?* (Wickham 2001) didn't make the Sunday Times bestseller list, but it did get me invited to speak at a few conferences around the world. I was asked to speak on other topics as well. I found I enjoyed researching birth-related questions and then teaching others about them, and I managed to dovetail that with my pre-existing love of research and statistics. My research on Anti-D was the catalyst for a career in birth information, writing and publishing on the side of my work as a midwife and lecturer.

Since that book, my first book, was published, I have authored or edited another fifteen books on different topics. Some of these have been updated several times when evidence, practice and thinking has changed. I have become aware over the past few years that I also needed to update my book on Anti-D, for much has changed in this area too. When I realised that 2021 marked the twentieth anniversary of the publication of the original book, it seemed fitting to mark the occasion with a new book.

I am sharing the story of my work in this area not just to introduce myself, or by means of explaining the significance of the publication date, but because it is key to how and why I have written and laid out this book. Thanks to the generosity of Elsevier, I have been able to incorporate the parts of the original text of *Anti-D in Midwifery: Panacea or Paradox?* that are still relevant into this book. But most of what is in this book is new; written with the benefit of twenty years of researching, speaking, writing and learning from women, families, midwives, doctors and others. I've learned quite a bit in the past two decades about the questions that people ask about Anti-D. In that time, there have also been changes in practice (e.g. when Anti-D is offered) and with the other tests and interventions that relate to this.

This edition of the book contains more information than the first book and it's written for those without prior knowledge. It has a new title and a new approach. I'm going to start by explaining the basics and then look at the evidence. My aim is to help readers who need to make decisions about this, as well as midwives, doctors, birth workers and others who would like to expand their knowledge. I've woven the story of my research through this book, as it's always more interesting to learn about research if it's told as part of a story of exploration than as a dull, dry series of facts. I have other stories to share, too: stories of conversations, stories of other research and stories of change, which show how we have moved on in some ways, and not at all in others.

There's another reason for telling my story at this point. I shared the note about needing to dig out dusty old medical journals in the era of web 1.0 to illustrate how important it is to remember how much the world has moved on in just a few decades. It's important to understand the history and context of what is happening now. This is true of so many areas, not just medical and maternity care. Most of the knowledge that modern maternity care is based on was developed in a context that was rather different to the context we live in today. One reason it's important to understand that is because we can't judge some things by today's standards. But this also begs important questions about the extent to which we're going to accept the status quo, or challenge it.

By raising questions about this area, I was not then and I am not now denying the life-saving nature of Anti-D. As one of the medical world's success stories, Anti-D has saved the lives of thousands of babies since its discovery and introduction. In fact, it was chosen by Time magazine as one of the top ten medical achievements of the 1960s. Few people would question the place of such a product in modern maternity care, or the importance of the work carried out in this area. Yet it is precisely because a few women were questioning their need for Anti-D that it seemed important to research this area be able to answer their questions. In order to make progress, we must sometimes ask questions that are uncomfortable. In fact, I would argue that the uncomfortable questions may be among the most important questions to ask.

What I didn't know when I first embarked on this research journey was that the story I would begin to uncover more than twenty years ago wasn't just about Anti-D. I didn't simply unearth a few facts that rounded out the information in the leaflet for the benefit of those in my care. I discovered a deeper story, about priorities, policies and politics. This was a story about a crossroads, and about which road was taken and which roads were not. A story which – as the title of my first book illustrated – contains paradoxes, some of which remain just as pertinent today.

On a personal level, that story has been the driving force behind much of the work that I have done since I first sat amongst the dusty bookshelves in Oxford, England. We have on the one hand created some amazing advances, while at the same time taken an approach which has not prioritised the ability of individuals to be able to make the decisions that are right for them. It's a story that needs to be told, and told again. I hope you'll enjoy it, and find it useful.

Sara Wickham. Wiltshire, England. Spring 2021.

1. Introducing the issues

In this chapter, I will explain the basics of this topic and a few of the terms that I use throughout the book. One key thing to know before we go too much further is that the term 'anti-D' refers to two different things. The first is a type of antibody that is naturally produced by the human body when the body encounters a particular substance. When I write about this kind of anti-D, I use a lower case 'a'. Anti-D is also the name of a type of medicine made from blood which contains this antibody and which is given to stop the human body from producing its own antibodies. I use a capital 'A' when I am talking about the medicine.

Every story has a location, and most of what happens in the story of anti-D (and Anti-D) takes place in an important bodily fluid: the blood. So that's where I'll begin. I'm going to repeat some of the key facts a few times in the first chapter or two. This is a complex area and I know people will dip in and out of this book. If you're familiar with the basics, please excuse the repetition and skip the bits you already know.

Blood, antigens and antibodies

Our blood, the fluid that is essential to life, and our hearts, which pump it around our bodies so that it can move all manner of other things between our cells, are so pivotal to our physicality that they are the stuff of poems and literature. Blood contains plasma and several different kinds of cells as well as all the substances that it transports, which include hormones, proteins, glucose, oxygen and carbon dioxide. It flows to nourish every part of our bodies, heals wounds, removes waste products, regulates our bodily systems and helps us to stave off and fight illness.

Blood has also long been the subject of medical study. Modern western medical knowledge has uncovered several differences between different people's blood. Some of these are categorised as being different blood types, and they are often grouped according to what kind of antigens a person's blood contains. Antigens are, of course, only one element of what is contained in a person's blood, but they are an important element as far as health care is concerned. That's because an antigen is a substance that can provoke an immune response and make the body produce antibodies. The 'job' of antibodies is to fight off the invading substance. We still have much to learn about antibodies, but the current thinking is that we are born with some antibodies, we gain some from our mother during birth and breastfeeding, and we develop others throughout our lives, for example if we encounter a foreign substance (perhaps naturally or through vaccination) and our body creates antibodies in response.

It's not as simple as saying that antigens are always 'bad' invaders and antibodies are always 'good' responders, though. It's true that antigens include toxins, bacteria and the viruses which cause colds, flu and worse. It's also true that antibody responses are generally marvellous and form the basis of good immunity, which is important for our survival. But the human antigen-antibody response doesn't always work to our advantage. Antigens also include, for instance, the cells of transplanted organs, which is why people who have organ transplants need to take drugs to suppress their immune systems. So there are situations – including the one we're going to look at throughout this book – where we don't always want a person's body to produce antibodies.

The most commonly known blood typing system is known as the ABO system, in which humans may have blood type A, B, AB or O. This system describes whether or not a person has one, both or neither of the A and B antigens in their blood. A person with blood type A just has the A antigen, a person with blood type B just has the B antigen, a person with blood type AB has both and a person with blood type O has neither.

As you may know, this becomes important if the person receives a blood transfusion. One reason it's important is that these are amongst the types of antibodies that we are born with. We don't want to give somebody blood from a person who has an antigen that they don't already have, as their antibodies can react with the antigen. In the worst case scenario, this can cause the donor blood cells to clump together (or agglutinate), which can interfere with blood flow. The donated blood cells may also haemolyse, which means that they split open and release haemoglobin into the body. Haemoglobin is the part of the blood that carries oxygen around the body and it is fabulous and essential to life when it is in the correct place. We don't want it outside of red blood cells though, as it is toxic in that situation. So it is of huge importance that, when giving someone donated blood, we make sure that it doesn't contain antigens that are going to cause a problem. Every time someone has a blood transfusion or an operation in which they might need blood, scientists in hospital laboratories carefully check the person's blood type and whether they have any antigens. They then cross-match the person's blood with donated blood that is available in the hospital so that the person will only receive donor blood that is compatible with their own blood.

The rhesus factor

There are other antigens that can either be present or absent in human blood and, although they are less well known than the A and B antigens, they are just as critical. The next most important blood group system (after the ABO system) is known as the rhesus factor system. The rhesus system currently contains more than 50 known antigens (Vege & Westhoff 2019) and this number may well increase as more are discovered. These include the rhesus factors c, C, D, e and E. The D antigen is considered the most important, because it is the most immunogenic, by which we mean the one most likely to produce an immune response (Choate 2018). For that reason, the terms 'rhesus positive' and 'rhesus negative' are often used to describe a person who either has or does not have the rhesus D factor in their blood. Although the correct term is rhesus D positive (or negative), I'm going to use the terms rhesus, rhesus negative and rhesus positive for ease of reading, so please assume from this point on that, when I write rhesus positive/negative, I am referring to the rhesus D factor unless I state otherwise.

If you have already had a blood test or donated blood, you may already know your rhesus group. Or perhaps (like me) you know because your mother was told your blood group after you were born. Whether or not we have this factor is genetically determined. The likelihood of someone being rhesus negative varies according to ethnicity. One per cent of people of Asian descent, eight per cent of people of African descent and 15 per cent of people of European descent are rhesus negative. The only way to determine whether an individual is rhesus positive or negative is by a blood test although, as I will describe in chapter two, it is now possible to tell whether an unborn baby is rhesus positive or negative by testing their mother's blood.

People who are rhesus positive are never compromised by their rhesus status. However, if a person who is rhesus negative comes into contact with the rhesus factor (for instance by receiving donated blood from a rhesus positive person), their blood will recognise the rhesus factor as foreign and produce antibodies to help remove it from their system. These antibodies remain in the body and enable the person to 'fight off' further rhesus factor in the future. That won't cause problems for most males. It doesn't usually pose a problem to a woman who is currently pregnant. It's also not an issue for a woman who isn't going to become pregnant in the future, even if she is currently pregnant. But it can be an issue for women who will have more babies in the future. That's because those antibodies can affect a future rhesus positive baby. Let's look at that in a bit more depth.

The rhesus factor and pregnancy

In pregnancy, the mother's and baby's blood does not usually mix. Their blood vessels are kept separate by means of an amazing pattern of structures within the placenta, which allows nutrients and oxygen to pass from the mother to the baby while at the same time allowing carbon dioxide and other waste products to be removed. But sometimes, either during pregnancy or around the time of birth, a small amount of the baby's blood enters the mother's bloodstream.

If the woman is rhesus positive, that's not a problem. If this happens in a rhesus negative woman whose baby is also rhesus negative, no adverse consequences will result, even if the ABO blood type is different. As I said above, the situation that causes concern is if the woman is rhesus negative and the baby is rhesus positive and some of the baby's blood enters the rhesus negative woman's bloodstream. We call this situation a fetomaternal transfusion. It's also known as a fetomaternal or transplacental haemorrhage, and is often abbreviated to FMH. Usually only a tiny amount of blood is involved though, and 'haemorrhage' does not mean a big loss of blood. It's usually less than a teaspoonful and it doesn't harm the baby. It can affect the woman's body though, as I have described. As a reminder, her blood may recognise the baby's blood as foreign and make anti-D antibodies. These antibodies won't hurt her, and they won't hurt her current baby, but the presence of the antibodies can be a problem if she later becomes pregnant with a rhesus positive baby. I'll describe the problem they cause below.

The process that I have just described (where the woman's blood makes antibodies to an antigen) is called a primary immune response. It leads to the production of a type of antibody called immunoglobulin M, or IgM antibodies. This process of producing IgM antibodies is known as sensitisation or isoimmunisation and it takes several days. These IgM antibodies don't stay in the body forever, though. Once the IgM antibodies have counteracted the antigen, the woman's body stops producing them. Cleverly, though, the body retains a memory of how to respond if it encounters the same antigen again. From a physiological perspective, that's a very sensible, smart mechanism. It stops us from passing the same cold viruses around forever. Once somebody has developed antibodies to an antigen, if the same antigen enters the body again, the body can mount what is known as a secondary immune response and quickly produce the antibodies (which it now knows how to make) and get rid of the invading substance. A secondary immune response usually occurs much faster than a primary immune response. The antibodies that it produces will come in a different form. This time, they are called immunoglobulin G or IgG.

I'd like to recap and put that into the context of explaining what can happen 'naturally' (that is, in a situation where we're not giving injectable Anti-D) if a rhesus negative woman encounters rhesus positive blood. When her blood detects the rhesus positive blood, her body may recognise the anti-D as an antigen. (I say 'may' here simply because we don't know if it always happens. We know it can happen, we know it does happen in some cases, but we don't know if it always happens. More on that in chapter four). When that happens, her body will mount a primary immune response and she would make IgM antibodies to the rhesus positive cells. Once the rhesus positive blood cells have all been cleared from her bloodstream, her antibody production will slow down and then stop. But her body will store that information and, over the next few weeks or months, will develop a 'template' for creating those antibodies. This is what has happened to someone who is described as sensitised or isoimmunised. In reality, the science is much more complex than this, but that is a quick overview of how we develop immunity.

Being sensitised (or isoimmunised) to anti-D can be a problem if a rhesus negative woman wants more babies in the future. If a sensitised woman later becomes pregnant with a rhesus positive baby, her body now knows how to recognise the D protein on a rhesus positive baby's blood cells and make IgG antibodies against that rhesus positive baby's blood. (Those antibodies wouldn't hurt or affect a rhesus negative baby). This is why women are offered an injection of the manufactured Anti-D medicine in situations where they might come into contact with their baby's blood. I'll discuss what those situations are in the next section. The manufactured Anti-D is said to "*...clear the fetal cells...*" (Qureshi *et al* 2014: 11). This is a slightly ambiguous phrase, and that's because we don't know exactly how Anti-D works to 'clear' those cells. In simple terms, manufactured Anti-D binds to blood cells with D on them and flags them up to a key part of the immune system which means that they are destroyed, before the part of the immune system that recognises the cells as foreign can kick in and make the antibodies (anti-D) that we don't want the woman to have. Throughout this book, I'm going to simply say that Anti-D clears fetal cells, rather than writing that out each time.

Even though we don't know exactly how Anti-D works, we know that it does work. Manufactured Anti-D effectively prevents the need for the woman's body to make natural anti-D antibodies. That means that any future rhesus positive babies the woman may become pregnant with are not at risk from those antibodies.

Why isn't the first/current baby affected?

There's a question I want to discuss in a bit more depth, because some people ask why the first rhesus positive baby born to a rhesus negative woman isn't usually affected by rhesus disease, even if she becomes sensitised during that pregnancy. Very occasionally, a woman's first baby *is* affected, but usually that's because she was sensitised before she became pregnant. And if that is the situation for you then you will find out as a result of the blood tests that all women are offered to check whether they are already sensitised in early pregnancy. More on those in chapter two. A very few women become sensitised before a first pregnancy from a previous mismatched blood transfusion, but this is extremely rare nowadays, especially in high-income countries. That's because we have been carefully typing and checking blood for a long time now. It is also possible for someone to become sensitised by injecting themselves using needles shared with others who have rhesus positive blood (Erickson 2020).

It's also theoretically possible, although also rare these days, especially given the modern focus on early pregnancy tests and fertility apps, that someone can be pregnant and lose a baby without realising. So they think they are pregnant with their first baby, but actually it's their second. There is some disagreement among organisations about the cut-off point at which Anti-D should be offered. In the UK, Anti-D is offered before 12 weeks of pregnancy only where there is an *"…ectopic pregnancy, molar pregnancy, therapeutic termination of pregnancy and in cases of uterine bleeding where this is repeated, heavy or associated with abdominal pain."* (Qureshi *et al* 2014). The Royal Australian and New Zealand College of Obstetricians and Gynaecologists (RANZCOG 2019) recommend that Anti-D is given no matter the situation or how early the gestation. The discrepancy most likely results from there being no robust evidence, as I discuss in chapter three.

But (some people then ask), could the baby that a woman is currently pregnant with (which may or not be her first) be affected if there is some kind of accident or intervention and their mother encounters their blood, say at 14 or 16 weeks? Could the mother become sensitised, develop the template to make antibodies and then pass them back to the same baby later in pregnancy? The answer to this is that it is indeed possible to become sensitised in pregnancy – and we will look at this in the chapter on giving Anti-D in pregnancy – but this would not affect the baby she was currently carrying. There are a couple of different reasons for this.

The first part of the reason that the current baby isn't affected by sensitisation during the pregnancy, is that IgM antibodies (which are the ones made during the primary response) are about six times bigger than the IgG antibodies that are made if a woman encounters rhesus positive blood for a second or subsequent time. This is important because IgG antibodies can cross the placenta, but IgM antibodies can't. So a woman who is mounting a primary immune response to rhesus positive blood cells is not going to be producing the kind of antibody that can cross the placenta to harm her growing baby, even if that baby is rhesus positive. But there's a second part to this. It takes some time to make the template. So unless the woman was sensitised before the pregnancy began (and has already had a primary response which means she has the template to make IgG antibodies), the baby that she is currently carrying is not at risk.

So Anti-D isn't given to protect the baby in the current pregnancy. It's all about protecting a woman's future babies. That makes it a really interesting situation, but it also means that anyone who is unsure about whether they want Anti-D can take their situation – that is, whether they might have more babies in the future – into account. We'll come back to this later. First, I want to explain what we're trying to prevent.

Rhesus disease

As we have seen, if a rhesus negative woman becomes pregnant with a rhesus positive baby and some of the baby's blood enters her bloodstream, she may become sensitised and develop the ability to make antibodies against the rhesus factor. As a result, any rhesus positive baby that she becomes pregnant with in the future may be affected. We use the term rhesus disease to describe a series of things that can happen if IgG antibodies enter the bloodstream of a rhesus positive baby. In simple terms, they can attack the rhesus proteins in the baby's blood. Rhesus disease is one of a group of diseases known as haemolytic disease of the fetus and newborn (HDFN). It may also be called Rh(D) disease but I use the simpler term 'rhesus disease' in this book.

Rhesus disease can impact the baby both before and after the birth, but in slightly different ways. When a baby develops rhesus disease in the womb, the main problems are anaemia and heart failure. Once the baby is born, jaundice may also be a problem. I am going to describe these processes in order to explain the problem, but please remember that they only affect a small number of babies. As I explain below, we can screen for and treat most babies with rhesus disease.

If anti-D antibodies attack the blood cells of a rhesus positive baby and begin to destroy their red blood cells, the concentration of red cells and the haemoglobin they contain begins to fall. This fall is what we are describing when we say someone has anaemia. Haemoglobin is the part of the red blood cell which carries oxygen around a person's body, so with fewer haemoglobin molecules, oxygen transport in the baby's body becomes harder.

To compensate for this, the baby increases their heart rate and changes where blood is moved around the body to help avoid damage to their cells from low oxygen levels. If the baby's haemoglobin levels continue to fall, the heart can reach a point where it is no longer able to function effectively. We call this heart failure although this term doesn't mean that the heart isn't working at all and that nothing can be done. Heart failure means that the heart isn't pumping as well as it should be. As a result, fluid can begin to accumulate in the baby's skin and around internal organs. This is known as ascites. Midwives and doctors also used the word 'hydrops' to describe what happens if a developing baby's organs can't overcome the anaemia that can occur in this situation.

Both the changes in blood flow and the accumulation of fluid can be seen on an ultrasound scan. If haemoglobin levels drop low enough, damage to the cells of the body begins to occur and death may occur. These days, rhesus disease is usually picked up and treatment begins well before this stage.

One treatment that has made a big difference in babies affected by rhesus disease is intrauterine transfusion (IUT). This treatment gives blood to the unborn baby through a needle inserted through the pregnant woman's abdomen and into a vessel in the umbilical cord. Ultrasound is used to help guide the needle into the correct place. In 2020, Tyndall *et al* reported that, *"Despite potential complications, overall survival rates have been reassuring since the early years of intravascular IUT, with reports of survival ranging from 82% to 96% in the years 1988 to 1997."* They concluded their paper by noting that, *"With access to current, expert surveillance and interventions for rhesus incompatible pregnancies, favourable outcomes for the fetus and neonate can be expected."* (Tyndall *et al* 2020: 5).

I noted that jaundice may also occur after birth in a baby who has rhesus disease, so I will explain how this happens too. All humans need red blood cells, but it is normal for such cells to only last for a few days, after which they get 'broken down' and sent to the liver in a sort of recycling process.

Jaundice happens when a baby is breaking down more red blood cells than its liver can manage. That might happen because the baby has a lot of red blood cells, or because its liver isn't yet fully coping with the demand, or both. It is common to see jaundice in a newborn baby; it often appears a couple of days after birth and it has usually gone in a week. But it can also appear when a baby is having a problem, such as rhesus disease. Again, treatment is available.

The word 'jaundice' itself describes how a baby's skin and the whites of their eyes can become yellow in colour. This is more noticeable in the skin of white babies. In dark skinned babies, jaundice can be seen in their eyes, on the palms of the hands and the soles of the feet. The yellowing is caused by the presence of a chemical called bilirubin. Bilirubin is a key by-product of the breakdown of red blood cells. Bilirubin readily crosses the placenta, so in pregnancy it is broken down in the mother's body. After birth, the baby has to break down and remove the bilirubin on its own. The baby's body does this by moving the bilirubin to just under the skin, where it can be broken down by light. This is why midwives have long suggested putting a slightly jaundiced baby outside, though not in direct sunlight, and it's also why the most common treatment for jaundice is to put a baby under a special kind of light, also called phototherapy.

If many red blood cells are being broken down at once (like in rhesus disease), then levels of bilirubin can rise quickly. Very high levels of bilirubin can cause permanent damage to brain tissue, in a condition known as kernicterus. This is very rare. NHS data show that this affects fewer than one in every 100,000 babies born in the UK (NHS 2021). A medical treatment called exchange transfusion is used to prevent damage from jaundice. This involves removing the baby's blood and replacing it with donated blood as the donated blood cells will not be affected by the anti-D antibodies.

Before Anti-D was available, rhesus disease affected one per cent of all newborns in populations of European descent and was responsible for the death of one baby in every 2,200 births (Kumar & Regan 2005). The Anti-D programme and related advances drastically reduced this. Many advances in the care of sick babies have also occurred over the past few decades. So it's hard to measure the exact contribution of each component. This in turn makes it hard to be clear on some of the numbers relating to the risks in this area, but we'll come back to that later in the book.

Sensitisation doesn't automatically mean that all of a woman's future babies will have rhesus disease. Subsequent rhesus negative babies will be unaffected by sensitisation, and some rhesus positive babies are also unaffected. Rhesus disease is mild in some affected babies and moderate or severe in others, but in its most severe form and without effective treatment it can be life-threatening or fatal. Thanks to advances in pregnancy and neonatal care as well as the widespread use of Anti-D, the number of babies who die from rhesus disease is now very small. In high-income countries, babies who are at risk of rhesus disease will be identified during the pregnancy blood tests offered to all rhesus negative women that I describe in chapter two. 'At risk' babies are identified when women are found to have antibodies, and you may hear or see this described as an antibody titre. The word titre (or titer, in the USA) simply means the concentration of something.

A proportion of women who are found to have rhesus antibodies (and unfortunately it is difficult to state exactly what proportion, because the data are not easily accessible) will have a low level of these, and their babies will be either unaffected or they may just have mild and easily treated jaundice. One of the reasons that we don't have good data on the frequency of this situation is that many of the women who have a low level of antibodies will have blood testing and other monitoring (such as ultrasound) during pregnancy, but they will remain in the care of their own midwife or doctor. They will not come to the attention of a specialist centre where data on treatments and outcomes are collected for research studies. Research midwife colleagues believe that we may have better information on this sort of thing in the future as data and medical notes become more digital.

We do have better data on the outcomes of the babies born to sensitised women who have high antibody titres and who receive specialist care and treatment as a result. We can see from the progression of research studies carried out over the years that the survival rate is increasing as knowledge grows and treatments get better. By 2008, more than 90% of the babies who were severely affected by rhesus disease survived (Smits-Wintjens & Lopriore 2008). Thanks to advances in neonatal intensive care, this number keeps increasing.

But these babies may need blood transfusions, early birth and/or intensive care and so there remains a big and important emphasis on preventing the problem of rhesus disease from occurring in the first place. It is also important to remember that, although it is not often the focus of research, the monitoring and treatment can be really stressful for both the baby and its parents, and even a 96% survival rate means that four per cent (or one in 25) of the babies severely affected by rhesus disease will not survive. Up to ten percent of those who survive severe rhesus disease may have long-term effects (Franklin 2009) and I want to finish this section by mentioning the one thing that always strikes me when I look at the studies and papers documenting the success of the Anti-D programme and the monitoring, treatment and outcomes of rhesus disease. That is, there is an almost complete lack of focus on parents' experiences, how those affected by the Anti-D programme, sensitisation and/or rhesus disease feel about this, or what their priorities are, or would be if they were only asked.

The permanence of sensitisation

One crucially important thing to know is that sensitisation is permanent. Forever. If someone becomes sensitised to an antigen, they will always be sensitised. This is such an important fact that I have given it its own section.

There are many situations in maternity care where it is possible to 'wait and see'. Some parents decide, for instance, to decline routine interventions and see how things go. That's because some interventions can be given later and still be beneficial. Or they can be given as a specific treatment (where they have the same beneficial effect) rather than as a preventative measure. One example of this, for instance, is the giving of an oxytocic drug for the birth of the placenta. These drugs can either be given as a preventative measure (in an attempt to reduce bleeding) or as a treatment, if too much blood is being lost (Edwards & Wickham 2018). So while there are situations in which a medically managed placental birth is undoubtedly a good idea, it's also sometimes possible to wait and see how things go before making a decision to accept a particular medicine or intervention (Wickham 2018a).

That's absolutely not the case with Anti-D. If you decline it and become sensitised, you can't decide to have it later and become 'unsensitised.' That's just not physically possible. You can't 'obliviate' your blood after the fact and make it forget how to make those antibodies. And (in contrast to the bleeding that can happen after birth) your midwife or doctor can't see whether any blood has passed from the baby's bloodstream into yours. Neither can any test that is currently available tell you if this has happened. We can do a test called a Kleihauer test, which I'll describe in the next chapter, but that only tells us if there is a lot of the baby's blood in the woman's bloodstream. There is no test that can detect a tiny amount, but even a tiny amount can cause sensitisation.

These are really important things to know. I don't tell you this to scare you into agreeing to have Anti-D at every opportunity, and there are many other aspects to this decision, but it would be very remiss of me not to mention this key fact in chapter one. The decision is always yours, no matter the intervention, medicine or treatment that is on offer. But it's not possible to wait and see if you become sensitised and then, if you do, to have Anti-D later and reverse the problem. We cannot undo sensitisation; we can only attempt to prevent it. And the only way we have of preventing it at this point in history is by the use of the manufactured form of Anti-D. So let's take a look at that.

Introducing Anti-D

I need to properly introduce the second type of Anti-D, and I've already noted that I'll be giving this a capital letter throughout the book to help you differentiate the two kinds. Because, as a quick recap, while the term anti-D can refer to the antibodies produced by the human body to fight off the rhesus D antigen, Anti-D is also the name of a manufactured substance that can be given as a prophylactic (preventative) treatment to prevent sensitisation from occurring. The antibodies in manufactured Anti-D clear the fetal blood cells and can prevent someone from making their own anti-D antibodies. Different doses of Anti-D are offered in different situations, depending on how much of the baby's blood is thought to have entered its mother's bloodstream.

Anti-D is a short way of describing a substance whose full name is Anti-D (Rho) Immunoglobulin. It's also called Rho(D) Immune Globulin, and different manufacturers use different brand names. In the UK, we use D-GAM® and Rhophylac® and the USA and some other countries use RhoGAM®. These are the same thing, although they come in different doses and different production standards are used around the world.

More on that in chapter two, when I will discuss the history and use of Anti-D, how it is made and possible side effects.

Although many people refer to Anti-D as a blood product, it's actually a medicine made from blood. It's a prescription medicine and it needs to be kept in a fridge in order to preserve its effectiveness. Anti-D is usually given by an injection into a muscle. It can be given into a vein or under the skin, for example if someone has a bleeding disorder. As you now know, its main action is to prevent the body from mounting a primary immune response to rhesus positive blood cells. This is beneficial because, if a woman mounts such a response and then later becomes pregnant with a rhesus positive baby, the effects of that immune response could lead to her producing IgG antibodies that could cross the placenta and harm a future rhesus positive baby.

Anti-D is truly one of the medical world's success stories, and I will be returning to tell more of the story about how it was discovered, developed and researched in chapters three and four. Before I do that, though, and because I know that many people want to know about the ins and outs of the various tests, treatments and interventions that are offered during pregnancy and childbirth, in chapter two I'm going to explain how, when and why Anti-D is offered, and the tests that relate to it.

2. Anti-D: when, why, how?

In this chapter, I'm going to give an overview of the care, tests and preventative treatments (Anti-D) that rhesus negative women are offered during pregnancy, birth and the postnatal period. I'm also going to answer some of the basic questions that people have about the Anti-D injection and discuss the side effects of this in women. There's a discussion about the side effects of Anti-D in relation to unborn babies in chapter three.

Today, as is so often the case in medical and maternity care, the exact recommendations relating to the offering of Anti-D and related tests differ according to where you are in the world. This illustrates the fact that debate is ongoing and there are still things we do not know about the ideal timing and dosages of Anti-D. But the principles, tests and timings are broadly similar around the world so, if you're thinking about your own options, this chapter is a good basis for a conversation with your care provider about what you will be offered in your area.

If you are rhesus negative and pregnant, your midwife or doctor should offer you information on Anti-D and on what tests are offered locally. This should happen at the beginning of pregnancy. If you haven't yet been given adequate information, you might want to ask for this, as there are both national and local variations. If you don't feel that the information you have been given is adequate, you are entitled to ask for more information. It is your right to decide whether you want to accept or decline Anti-D. It is also your right to request Anti-D, even if someone isn't offering it. You may or may not be entitled to get it, but it doesn't hurt to ask. If you are told that you are not able to have Anti-D, someone should explain to you why this is, and what other options you have.

When and why is Anti-D offered?

In general, there are two broad recommendations about when Anti-D should be offered to rhesus negative women in current maternity care. The first recommendation – at least in most high-income countries – is that Anti-D should be offered within 72 hours of any potentially sensitising event, or PSE. A PSE is any event that might be associated with a baby's blood entering its mother's bloodstream. The most important of these is giving birth to a rhesus positive baby, but they also include other situations.

Below, I share a list by Qureshi *et al* (2014) of the PSEs for which Anti-D is offered in the UK. I want to acknowledge that it contains some medical terms which relate to situations, tests and interventions which might not be instantly understood by the lay person. In general, the list includes any situation in which a baby is born; in which there is bleeding (PV bleeding means bleeding from the vagina); in which damage may have occurred to the placenta (either by accident or as the result of medical intervention); or in which a baby sadly dies during pregnancy. The terms in this list of PSEs are all searchable online if you would like more detail, and the list includes:

*"Amniocentesis, chorionic villus biopsy and cordocentesis
Antepartum haemorrhage/uterine (PV) bleeding in pregnancy
External cephalic version
Abdominal trauma (sharp/blunt, open/closed)
Ectopic pregnancy
Evacuation of molar pregnancy
Intrauterine death and stillbirth
In-utero therapeutic interventions (transfusion, surgery, insertion of shunts, laser)
Miscarriage, threatened miscarriage
Therapeutic termination of pregnancy
Delivery – normal, instrumental or Caesarean section
Intra-operative cell salvage."* (Qureshi *et al* 2014).

It's important to know that the 72 hour timeframe is not an absolute cut-off point. It was the timeframe used in the early studies, some of which were conducted among prisoners (most famously in Sing Sing Prison), where logistics decreed that the Anti-D was given within 72 hours of the rhesus negative subject being injected with rhesus positive blood (Romm 1999). We now know that Anti-D can be effective if given up to ten days after a potentially sensitising event (Qureshi *et al* 2014). But sooner is better, not least because, if this is left until later, especially where care is fragmented and you don't always see the same midwife or doctor each time, there is more chance that it will be forgotten.

The second situation in which Anti-D is recommended in many high-income countries is as a routine precaution during pregnancy for all rhesus negative women. There is more variation and more controversy around this recommendation than around the idea that we should offer Anti-D after a PSE. I'm going to look at the history and the evidence for both of these situations in chapter three.

Who doesn't need Anti-D?

It's also important to know who doesn't need Anti-D. As you now know from chapter one, Anti-D doesn't protect the current baby. That's because the current baby doesn't need protection. If the current baby is rhesus negative, it can't be harmed by anti-D antibodies. But even if the current baby is rhesus positive, *unless the mother is sensitised before pregnancy begins* (and I'll explain more about how we can find that out below), antibody production wouldn't happen in time to harm it before it was born. I explained this in some depth in chapter one. Sensitisation wouldn't affect any future rhesus negative babies either. Anti-D is given only for the benefit of possible future rhesus positive babies.

This is actually quite an unusual situation as far as medical care goes. It is one of the reasons that my first book on this subject was subtitled *'panacea or paradox?'* One of the key paradoxes is that Anti-D is the only medical treatment that I know of about which the following three things can be said:

(1) It is given to a person (the mother) who doesn't physically benefit from it.
(2) When it is given in pregnancy, it is given to the possible detriment of another person who won't physically benefit from it. By this we mean the unborn baby. This is because of the chance of side effects on the baby, which I look at in chapter three. This doesn't apply when Anti-D is given after the birth of a baby, although (1) and (3) still apply in that situation.
(3) It is given for the possible benefit of a person who does not yet exist and who may never exist.

None of that is to take away from everything I said in the previous chapter about how amazing Anti-D is, but it does make one think.

With this in mind, because Anti-D is only given for the benefit of future rhesus positive babies, if someone is certain that they won't be having any more babies in the future, then they may not wish to have Anti-D. In some areas, women who are going to have a tubal ligation or other procedure for permanent contraception during or after birth will be told that they do not need Anti-D, and this applies to Anti-D which might be offered at any point during pregnancy as well.

The second situation in which Anti-D isn't necessary is if you know for sure that the baby you are carrying is rhesus negative. There are two possible ways that you might know this. One is when the results of antenatal rhesus testing or non-invasive prenatal testing (NIPT) show that the baby is rhesus negative, and I will explain these tests later in this chapter. Or you may know for certain that the father of the baby is rhesus negative. When two rhesus negative people have a baby together, the baby can only be rhesus negative, so in this situation Anti-D will not be needed during pregnancy, birth or afterwards. There's a small section on genetics in chapter five if you would like an overview of this.

If you are certain that the baby's father is rhesus negative, and you raise it as a reason to want to decline Anti-D, don't be surprised if a health care provider questions you on this, or wants to talk to you about it alone. It can be really annoying to be questioned in this way, I know, and people sometimes feel cross if they are treated as if they may not be telling the truth about whether their partner is the father of their baby (Plested & Kirkham 2016).

From the perspective of those who are providing professional care, as you now know, one of the key issues is that sensitisation is irreversible. Care providers have a legal duty to check that anyone seeking care is fully aware of all aspects of their decisions. Midwives and doctors are only too aware that some women are living in violent or difficult situations which mean they feel unable to be honest in front of whoever is at the appointment with them. Midwives and doctors also know that some women feel unable to tell the truth (for instance if their partner is not the father of their baby) because they are worried that something will be written in their notes, which others may read later. So questioning about paternity happens not just to annoy or doubt you, but also because a caring health professional wants to be certain that you are not being coerced into saying something that isn't true. It's not personal. Annoying as it can be, it's usually done out of concern for your and others' wellbeing. That's not to say that coercion doesn't happen around Anti-D. It does. I'm just saying that double checking claims about paternity is often done with good intent, and because home is not a safe place for everyone.

That aside, it can also be frustrating that some health authorities and professionals ask for evidence that the baby's father is rhesus negative. It is up to you whether you provide them with this or not because, at the end of the day, it's your decision as to whether or not you have Anti-D. You're not legally obliged to provide proof or to satisfy anyone else of the 'reasonableness' of your decision. As long as you are an adult with capacity, you don't need anybody's permission to decline Anti-D or any other medical treatment. But, given the potential repercussions of being sensitised, which cannot be reversed, you might want to double check the baby's father's blood group and ask for help if you are unsure. There is more information on how to find out somebody's rhesus group in the frequently asked questions in chapter five.

Early pregnancy and blood tests

All women are offered a blood test in early pregnancy in order to determine their blood group and rhesus status and to help their midwife or doctor get a general view of their health. A sample of blood is taken from your arm, using a needle and syringe. You can ask what they are screening for and say if you do not want all or any of the tests. These blood tests are sometimes called 'booking bloods', or you might hear people talking about an 'FBC' (full blood count), 'CBC' (complete blood count) or 'Rh testing' (rhesus group testing).

This is the stage where a midwife or doctor will usually discover or confirm that a woman is rhesus negative, and all rhesus negative women will then be offered interventions which I shall describe throughout this chapter. But rhesus testing is just one of a number of tests that are done at this stage of pregnancy. Early pregnancy blood tests will also look for things like iron deficiency and certain diseases, such as HIV and hepatitis B or C. Your blood will be tested to see if you already have antibodies that could potentially cause a problem to you or your baby. As I explained in chapter one, there are other antigens that people can be sensitised to, and your blood test might show these, even if you are rhesus D positive. Be aware that not all of the antibodies that can be detected by this test are 'clinically significant.' That means that some of them would not pose a problem to your baby, so if you are told that you have antibodies then make sure you talk to a midwife or doctor about what that actually means for you and your baby.

If any antibodies (rhesus D or otherwise) are found which might pose a problem to a woman or baby, specialist care and monitoring will be offered, often including additional ultrasound tests. This is to monitor the situation and the baby so that treatment can be offered if there is concern about the baby. Because this is a rare situation and the treatment is highly specialised, affected women may be referred to a specialist centre, and these are often in large cities. In my experience, the midwives, doctors, scientists and nurses who work in such centres are highly knowledgeable and really good at explaining people's individual situations to them.

I have been stating that these blood tests are 'offered' in the paragraphs above but, in reality, most people go along with whatever tests are standard and do not tend to ask questions. Many people don't even realise that all medical tests and treatments are optional, and not all health care professionals present them as such. Some health professionals will tell you that you must have a particular test, although this is not true. They can advise it, but it's always up to you whether you have it or not. So sometimes blood testing is done without much discussion of the test or its consequences or the pros and cons of having it. Some people don't realise what they are being tested for. You should also always be advised of the results of any test, but we know that this doesn't always happen in practice. My advice, whether or not you are pregnant, is that, if any health professional wants to take blood, ask what it's for, how you will be informed of results and what the consequences of the results might be. One key question to ask is whether the results of the test might limit your options in any way. You don't have to agree to any test that you don't want, and you always have the right to ask for more information, to say no or to take time to consider whether it is right for you.

Informed consent and Anti-D

If blood testing shows that a woman is rhesus negative, she should be told this and given information about Anti-D and the pros and cons of having this in different situations so that she can make her own decision ahead of time. It is quite reasonable for someone to decide that they would want Anti-D in some situations but not others.

Most countries have clear guidelines (at least in theory) on informed consent and Anti-D. Here is the UK version:

"All pregnant women must be offered written and verbal information about anti-D Ig to inform their decision about receiving anti-D Ig. Maternal consent must be obtained prior to giving anti-D Ig, and the woman's decision to either accept or decline the injection should be clearly recorded by the healthcare professional, both in the woman's 'hand held' and hospital records (RCOG, 2011). NICE guidance recommends that choice is offered at the time of recording blood group in her antenatal healthcare records." (Qureshi *et al* 2014).

Again, this discussion may or may not happen. Some women report that they received good information and had an opportunity to ask questions. One said:

"It was great, actually. I had a leaflet and the chance to talk it through before I decided, and I was happy to have it."

36

Some say that they first they knew of Anti-D was when someone approached them with an injection.

"I was just told that I had a blood group which meant I would have to have injections. I don't know why."

Some felt that they were persuaded into it, and only later (in this case after encountering my work on this topic) did they question it:

"I was just given Anti-D at my 29 week appointment; I was reluctant because I didn't know what it was for, but the midwives were very persuasive."

It's not okay that this variability exists, but it would be remiss of me to pretend that it doesn't. It's not okay that many of the parents I talk to feel they have to inform and advocate for themselves, but that is also the reality, especially for those who do not want to take the standard path. Bureaucratic systems clearly need to have standards and guidelines so that they can function effectively, but flexibility is important as well. The existence of a guideline or standard offer doesn't mean that everybody has to accept everything they are offered. If you'd like to know more about that, please see my book, *'What's Right For Me?'* (Wickham 2018a).

Antenatal rhesus group testing

In the past few years, a new type of antenatal screening test has been developed and launched in several countries. This test is known as fetal RhD genotyping and it can show whether an unborn baby is rhesus positive or rhesus negative from a test performed on its mothers blood. A number of studies have showed that this test is feasible and that the false negative rate is extremely low, at 0.2% (Finning *et al* 2008, Manzanares *et al* 2014, de Haas *et al* 2016, Vivanti *et al* 2016).

No test is right all the time but that figure shows that this test is very accurate. In fact, if a rhesus negative woman has this test, is told that her baby is rhesus negative and decides not to have routine antenatal Anti-D as a result, her chances of becoming sensitised are only one in 86,000. When we take into account the fact that the chance of silent sensitisation is low, and that Anti-D itself is not 100% effective (although it is close), it is understandable that some countries – for example Denmark and The Netherlands – are offering rhesus group testing to all rhesus negative pregnant women so as to reduce the number of women unnecessarily exposed to Anti-D during their pregnancy.

Antenatal rhesus group testing may be offered as a single test (where the baby's rhesus group is the only thing that is being looked for) or as part of a more extensive type of screening test called NIPT, or non-invasive prenatal testing. Rather than write everything out twice, I'm going to move on to talk about NIPT, as this is the test that most readers of this book will encounter, but I'll note in the next section where the issues are similar and/or different for those who are offered antenatal rhesus group testing as a single test.

Non-invasive prenatal testing (NIPT)

Non-invasive prenatal testing (NIPT) is also a type of blood test carried out on a pregnant woman's blood. Like all tests, it's not perfect, but in some situations it can give us better information than previously available tests could but without performing a procedure which carries a risk to the baby. That's why it's called non-invasive.

The NIPT test, which you may also hear or see referred to as cell free DNA, cfDNA or chromosomal testing, looks for cells from the baby which have entered the blood of its mother. This is also the case where a blood test is being performed simply for antenatal rhesus group testing. It is usual for some tiny cells from the baby to enter its mother's bloodstream during pregnancy. These cells aren't generally blood cells which can cause the woman to form antibodies. The DNA from these fetal (baby) cells can be analysed and it can tell us certain things about the unborn baby. But where the antenatal rhesus group test simply looks for the baby's blood group, NIPT testing includes screening tests for other things as well. Like some other pregnancy screening tests, NIPT can give us an estimate of the chance that a baby has certain chromosomal anomalies or conditions, such as Down syndrome, and it can also determine the baby's sex.

Knowing whether the unborn baby is rhesus negative can be very helpful for those who are rhesus negative themselves. Let's imagine that a woman of European descent knows from a blood test that she is rhesus negative. If her partner is also of European descent (and I am using people of European descent in the example only because they have the highest chance of being affected by this issue), there is about a 42% chance that her baby is also rhesus negative, which means she won't need Anti-D at any point during that pregnancy or after the baby's birth. So it could be really helpful to know the baby's rhesus group, and this means that four in ten of the women in this situation won't need any Anti-D.

Having this sort of knowledge wasn't an issue when Anti-D was only offered after a baby was born, because we could test the baby's blood and find out if it was rhesus positive or negative before Anti-D was offered (or not). But it is very much an issue now that Anti-D is offered routinely in pregnancy as well as in response to PSEs. As a reminder, this is because women who are pregnant with a rhesus negative baby aren't at any risk of becoming sensitised. So, where we are offering Anti-D in pregnancy but don't know the blood group of the baby, a lot of Anti-D is given unnecessarily to women whose babies are rhesus negative.

A proportion of those women who access rhesus group testing, whether as a stand-alone test or as part of NIPT, will learn that their unborn baby is rhesus negative. Those women don't then even have to consider whether they want Anti-D in pregnancy, either routinely or after a PSE. They'll know from early on that they don't need it. Those who learn that their baby is rhesus positive can then decide what they want to do in regard to having Anti-D when it is offered or not; they also have more certainty.

The exact timing of rhesus group testing varies between countries and regions. It needs to be done late enough to have a good chance of being successful (because the baby sheds more cells as it grows, which makes the test easier to perform), but early enough to prevent unnecessary Anti-D being offered in the meantime. The past few years have seen a marked increase in the success of this test and it may become an option for more women over the next few years.

There are a few more things to know about NIPT, which is a more complex area than simple rhesus group testing. It is carried out between 11 and 16 weeks of pregnancy, and the optimal timing of NIPT may depend not just on issues relating to determining rhesus group (which isn't usually seen as the main point of NIPT testing) but also on whether the woman/family want other tests. NIPT is not yet available in all areas, or for everybody. It is not yet a standard part of care in all countries and, in some areas where it is available, those who want to use it may need to pay for it. One big advantage is that NIPT is far safer than invasive tests such as amniocentesis or chorionic villus sampling, which involve putting needles through the woman's abdomen and taking cells from the amniotic fluid or placenta. These invasive tests carry a risk of miscarriage.

But all tests have downsides and possible ramifications as well as advantages. NIPT is a highly accurate form of testing which has been developed over the past decade or so and which has been hailed around the world as a great breakthrough (Zhu *et al* 2014, Teitelbaum *et al* 2015, Neovius *et al* 2016, Vivanti *et al* 2016, de Haas *et al* 2016). But it isn't without limitations, just like all tests. As Uldbjerg (2017) discusses, the sensitivity of NIPT testing when it is used to look for chromosomal abnormalities is more than 99%. This means that in more than 99% of the cases where the baby does actually have a condition, this will be picked up by NIPT. However, Uldbjerg (2017) also showed that when NIPT is used in younger women who do not have risk factors, the positive predictive value is only 50%. This means that only in about half of the results that suggest that a baby might have a particular chromosomal anomaly does the baby actually have an anomaly. So if parents want to know for sure whether their baby has a chromosomal anomaly, they will still need an invasive diagnostic test (Uldbjerg 2017).

With NIPT, it's also important to know that there is always a chance of getting something called a 'no-call' result. This is what it is called when the NIPT fails to give a result, and it usually happens when there weren't enough fetal cells in the blood sample to be able to measure. This is more common when the woman weighs more than average (Uldbjerg 2017, Juul *et al* 2020), but it can also happen when certain conditions or abnormalities are present (Chan *et al* 2017, Uldbjerg 2017). Although none of these things relate directly to decisions about rhesus group testing and Anti-D, they are important to know about, as I will explain below.

As above, simple rhesus group testing is highly accurate. When it comes to the accuracy of NIPT in determining a baby's rhesus group, data analysed by NICE (2016) show that this is also very accurate.

"NIPT for fetal RHD genotype is very accurate among women with a rhesus-D (D) positive fetus; only 2 to 4 in 1,000 such women

will have a negative test result and so be at risk of sensitisation because they would not be offered antenatal anti-D immuneglobulin. NIPT for fetal RHD genotype is slightly less accurate among women with a D-negative fetus; between 13 and 57 in 1,000 such women will have a positive test result and so be offered antenatal anti-D immunoglobulin unnecessarily." (NICE 2016: section 4.3)

It can be quite complex to navigate NIPT and make sense of the information involved in such testing, and there are quite a lot of factors to take into account when deciding whether to have it. A key consideration, as I mentioned above, is whether you want all of the information that the NIPT would offer. NIPT is used mainly to look for chromosomal issues, including Down syndrome. It may or may not be possible to find out your baby's rhesus group without also finding out (or having someone else find out) your baby's sex or their chance of having a chromosomal issue.

If you are offered NIPT, ask what will be screened for, whether you can choose what is screened for and what the accuracy of each part of the test is likely to be. It is always worth thinking beforehand about the different results that you might get and what your options, feelings and desires would be in each situation. More information isn't always better. Sometimes, information can be an unwanted burden, or lead to painful decisions that can make people wish they hadn't had the test in the first place. So, as with any screening test, it's important to be sure you have full information about the pros and cons and a chance to think it through before deciding if it is right for you.

This is an area in which our knowledge is certain to grow and change over the next few years. That's partly because much of what I am writing about in this section is based on very recent research, and a number of key studies are ongoing. Many countries and regions are in the process of reconsidering guidelines and what is available and offered in different situations. There is wide variation in this area, so if you are pregnant or planning a pregnancy, you may want to find out what is currently available, and whether you will need to pay extra if you decide to have this. You may want to consider the chances of a 'no-call' result and ask what would happen in this situation.

Anti-D in pregnancy

There are two situations in which you might be offered Anti-D in pregnancy, which we also sometimes refer to as antenatal Anti-D. First, you should be offered antenatal Anti-D if you experience a PSE, or potentially sensitising event. Such events might include a car accident or fall in which you might have bumped your abdomen, vaginal bleeding after 12 weeks of pregnancy or a medical intervention that increases the chance of the baby's blood mixing with yours. I gave the full list of situations that are considered to be potentially sensitising events near the beginning of this chapter. But even if you do not experience any of these, in many countries all rhesus negative women are now offered one or two doses of Anti-D during pregnancy as a routine precaution. We sometimes refer to this as 'routine antenatal Anti-D'.

As I am going to discuss the evidence relating to the different timings of when we offer Anti-D in chapter three, I'm not going to list all of the pros and cons of routine antenatal Anti-D here. However, a significant part of the debate about routine antenatal Anti-D which I will discuss in more depth later in the book is that we know that, in reality, women are not always offered Anti-D after a potentially sensitising event. If they were, it is possible that routine antenatal Anti-D might not be needed. So, if you are rhesus negative and you know that you would want to have Anti-D after a PSE, it's important to (a) know what a PSE is and the different situations in which you might want Anti-D, and (b) contact your midwife or doctor as soon as possible after a PSE so that Anti-D can be given to you. If you are away from home when a PSE occurs and you're not due back within the next day or so, contact or visit the nearest hospital and tell them you want to discuss Anti-D. Depending on where you are in the world, you may need to ask to speak to a midwife or obstetrician, so don't be afraid to do that if you don't immediately get a positive response.

Some people feel that, in an ideal world, you should not have to be responsible for these things. I totally understand that argument. But sometimes people see a different midwife or doctor, or their notes go missing, or they have an accident while they are away from home and the person treating them isn't able to access their maternity care record. A story that I have heard a few times is that someone is on holiday, and they visit the local emergency department because they have been in a car accident or have some bleeding. No-one mentions or offers Anti-D, so they assume they don't need it. But later, they find that they have become sensitised.

In this situation, the Anti-D should have been offered in response to the PSE. But perhaps the person they saw in the emergency department didn't have enough experience of maternity care to think about this. Maybe it wasn't available locally, or an incorrect assumption was made that the woman would already have had routine antenatal Anti-D and that this would be enough. Maybe the country visited doesn't have enough Anti-D to offer it to visitors, or they don't offer it in that situation. There are many reasons that this kind of omission happens, and I'll return to this in chapter three. My point here is simply to recommend that you remain alert and always ask if you think you may benefit from having Anti-D. These days, even if you are far from home, you can usually contact your own midwife and, if it's appropriate and the timing works, they can have Anti-D ready for your return.

Anti-D after birth

As I will explain more fully in the next chapter, we know that some rhesus negative women who give birth to a rhesus positive baby will become sensitised if they do not have Anti-D after giving birth. So this is a key focus for midwives and doctors, and all rhesus negative women who give birth to a rhesus positive baby will be offered Anti-D within 72 hours of giving birth.

In most areas of the world, all rhesus negative women are offered a blood test for their baby just after birth which will find out their rhesus group. If a woman has had antenatal rhesus testing or NIPT (as described above), if the baby's father is known to be rhesus negative or in situations where genetic information is available, parents and care providers may already know the rhesus status of the baby. But many national guidelines suggest checking the baby's blood group anyway, in a 'better safe than sorry' approach. This is an area that may change over the next few years because of the high level of accuracy of rhesus group and NIPT testing.

The blood test is carried out on a sample of the baby's blood taken from the umbilical cord (if the mother agrees, of course) after the baby is born. It is perfectly possible and reasonable to ask the midwife or doctor to wait before doing this, especially if you want to have optimal cord clamping and/or a physiological placental birth (see Edwards & Wickham 2018 for more on this). There is no reason to need to clamp and cut the cord more quickly simply because a woman is rhesus negative. The blood that circulates between the baby and the placenta is what we call a closed system. In the first minutes after birth, the baby is adapting to life outside the womb and shifting blood to different areas around their body. There is good evidence to suggest that it is preferable to not clamp and cut the cord early, as this interferes with the baby's ability to take as much blood from the placenta as it needs (Edwards & Wickham 2018). There is no evidence that the baby's blood is more likely to get into the mother's bloodstream if we wait longer. In fact, some midwives have speculated that, by waiting and allowing the placenta to detach naturally, we may decrease the chance of fetomaternal transfusion (Wickham 2001) but no studies have been done to test this. I will discuss that theory a bit further in chapter four.

If the woman wants to wait and leave the cord unclamped for a while, the midwife or doctor can (with her consent) either take blood from the placenta (if it has been born) or from a vessel in the unclamped umbilical cord. There is some conversation amongst holistic midwives about whether it might be better to use one of the two umbilical arteries for this rather than the umbilical vein as (unlike everywhere else in the adult body) the arteries take blood away from the baby. We have no evidence that this makes a difference but the theory is that this may be less likely to interfere with the baby getting its full complement of blood than if the larger umbilical vein is used. If blood is taken from the unclamped cord then the midwife or doctor may need to put a little bit of pressure on the place where the needle went in to prevent bleeding. In the unlikely scenario that a sample cannot be obtained from the cord or placenta, it can be taken from the baby. This is also sometimes necessary if the blood sample from the cord is later found to be inadequate by the laboratory. Fear of another sample being needed is not a good reason to clamp the cord early. Later cord clamping is beneficial and another blood sample is occasionally needed even if the cord is clamped immediately.

Within about an hour after birth (but it will depend a bit on where you are), a sample of blood is also taken (again, only if consent is given) from the mother. Both blood samples are labelled and sent to the laboratory. Because laboratories are full of medical scientists who understand the issues relating to rhesus disease, this testing is usually prioritised and the results come back more quickly than for some other tests.

If the test on the cord blood shows that the baby is rhesus negative, no further testing is needed and there is no need to offer Anti-D. If the baby is found to be rhesus positive, then another test is done on the blood that was taken from the mother just after the birth. This sample is used to check for the presence of a fetomaternal transfusion, a test also known as a Kleihauer test. I'm going to talk about Kleihauer tests and the optimal doses of Anti-D in the next section, so for now I will simply say that this test is done to ensure that the correct amount of Anti-D is given. The tests will be done and, in most areas, the same laboratory will determine the necessary dose of Anti-D and send this to the woman's care provider so it can be given as soon as possible after birth. In many cases, this happens within a day of the birth, but the standard that most areas adhere to is that it should be given within 72 hours.

Once the correct dose of postnatal Anti-D has been offered/given (and more on the detail of that below as well), nothing more will happen (at least as far as Anti-D-related issues are concerned) until or unless the woman becomes pregnant again. Then, all of this will be repeated in her next pregnancy, beginning with the booking bloods to see if she has any antibodies, which does occasionally happen even when Anti-D is given and everything is done to the letter. In most cases though, if all of this happens at the right time, the Anti-D programme effectively prevents sensitisation, and we'll look at the evidence for that in the next chapter. But at the beginning of this paragraph I mentioned the idea of a 'correct dose' of Anti-D, and I need next to explain what that means and how we know how much Anti-D to offer each woman. Because a small number of women are found to need more than the standard dose of Anti-D when their blood is tested after birth.

Fetomaternal transfusion and Kleihauer testing

Anti-D comes in different doses, and each dose will clear a certain amount of fetal blood from the maternal circulation. A dose of 500iu (where iu stands for international units) of Anti-D is said to clear a fetomaternal bleed of up to 4ml. This is considered by some as a 'standard dose', but closer inspection reveals some variation, both in theory and practice.

The UK guidelines recommend that *"...at least 500iu..."* of Anti-D is given as the standard postnatal dose (Qureshi *et al* 2014: 9), but some areas give 500iu of Anti-D as a standard dose and others give 1500iu. In Australia and New Zealand, however, the standard dose recommended by RANZCOG (2019) is 625iu. Midwives and doctors in those countries also report that the actual dose given may differ from this.

In many countries, Anti-D is also available in smaller doses of 250iu for giving in pregnancy, when the amount of blood in a fetomaternal bleed would be smaller because the baby is smaller. The smallest dose of 250iu is called a micro dose or, in the USA, MICRhoGAM®. And, as well as being used as a standard dose in some parts of the world, the larger 1500iu dose of Anti-D is also used for when more than a standard dose of Anti-D is deemed to be necessary. This can happen when a larger fetomaternal transfusion is thought to have occurred.

Despite this variation (which I'll discuss further in chapters three and four), the standard dose of 500iu of Anti-D is considered the minimum amount for most women after giving birth. That's because very little (if any) of the baby's blood enters their circulation. But, because Anti-D is given to clear fetal blood cells, a woman who has more than 4ml of her baby's blood in her bloodstream needs more than a standard 500iu dose of Anti-D.

We think that a fetomaternal transfusion of more than 4ml happens in about one in a thousand cases (Moise 2002) but, as fetomaternal bleeding can be caused by some medical interventions, the chance of this happening may depend on where and how you give birth. Again, we can't see that a fetomaternal bleed has occurred by looking at someone, so we need a way of determining which women have experienced this, so that we can give them more Anti-D to clear the rest of the fetal blood. Otherwise the first dose of Anti-D will have been given in vain, because their body might still produce antibodies. It's a crude analogy, I know, but it's like throwing a teaspoonful of salt onto a whole glass of red wine that has spilled on the carpet. You might soak up a bit of the wine but there will still be a stain on the carpet. If you want to soak it all up, you need to pour on enough salt. One could even say that, if you're not going to pour on enough salt, you may as well not pour on any, but the difference between the wine in my analogy and the fetal blood that may be in a woman's bloodstream is that we can easily see how much wine is there.

So scientists have developed a test to check that we are giving enough Anti-D in a situation where we think a fetomaternal bleed might have occurred. It's called a Kleihauer test, and it is a widely available, slightly crude but also quite helpful way of estimating whether more than 4ml of fetal blood might have entered the mother's bloodstream. Kleihauer testing isn't used when giving routine Anti-D in pregnancy. But Kleihauer testing is widely available and it's the test most often used in conjunction with giving Anti-D after birth, after a road traffic accident, after a medical intervention in pregnancy and so on.

The Kleihauer test – which is also known as the Kleihauer–Betke or acid elution test - involves taking a drop of maternal blood and using a process (actually an acid bath and then the addition of a special dye, if you're interested) which makes the maternal haemoglobin disappear but leaves the fetal haemoglobin a rose pink colour. The operator smears a small sample of the blood onto a slide, examines it through a microscope, and counts the number of darker fetal cells that are visible. That number is used to estimate the total amount of fetal cells that may have entered the woman's bloodstream. If the Kleihauer test shows that more of the baby's blood cells have entered the maternal circulation than the standard dose of Anti-D that is given locally can clear, a higher dose of Anti-D will be offered. That's because it will take more Anti-D to clear a larger amount of fetal cells.

It's important to know that the Kleihauer test is not a test to see if there has been *any* fetomaternal bleeding. It is a screening test for a larger fetomaternal bleed than can be cleared by the standard dose of Anti-D. This is a really important distinction. If a woman has a negative Kleihauer test, it does not mean that there is no fetal blood in her circulation. There may be no fetal blood in her circulation, but the Kleihauer test isn't sensitive enough to tell us that. A really important thing to know is that laboratory scientists don't usually *expect* to see fetal blood on a Kleihauer test.

"If I see fetal blood..." one British scientist told me, *"...then that means the woman had a large transplacental haemorrhage and we'll be sending a bigger dose of Anti-D."*

All that a negative Kleihauer test can tell us is that no fetal blood can be seen, not that there isn't any in the maternal circulation. The reason this is important (and frustrating) is that sometimes, when people hear about the Kleihauer test, they think it might be a way to determine whether or not any fetomaternal bleeding has occurred, and thus as a way of determining that they can decline Anti-D, but it isn't. If you'd like an analogy to help make sense of that, imagine putting five small plastic ducks into a bath full of water and then closing your eyes and taking a scoop of water out with a tea cup. You might get a duck in your cup, but it's not very likely.

They're still there in the bath though. Now imagine tipping fifty ducks onto the water and scooping up another cupful of water. You're much more likely to get at least one duck in your cup that time. Just like the Kleihauer test, the 'tea cup test' can't tell you for certain that there are no ducks, but it will tell you if there is likely to be a large duck (or fetal blood cell) population in there.

So if the Kleihauer test is negative, we know that, even if there is a bit of fetal blood in the woman's circulation, this is likely to be an amount that can be cleared by the standard dose of Anti-D. If the result of the Kleihauer test on a woman's blood comes back positive then she will be offered additional doses of Anti-D. Scientists may also use a test called flow cytometry, which enables them to more accurately estimate the volume of fetal blood that has entered the maternal circulation. But whichever test is used, the dosage of Anti-D will be carefully calculated by haematologists and a woman in this situation will be offered larger doses of Anti-D and repeat testing until no more fetal blood can be seen (Qureshi *et al* 2014).

There are conditions, notably an inherited blood disorder called beta thalassaemia, that can lead to a false positive Kleihauer result. These conditions affect only a tiny number of people and the routine blood tests offered during pregnancy in many countries include a test for the gene that causes this condition.

I will return to a discussion of dosage in the next chapter, when I will look at the evidence relating to Anti-D. First I'd like to address the practical questions of how Anti-D is made and given and then outline the side effects and some of the concerns that midwives and parents have raised.

How is Anti-D made?

Often, people ask about how Anti-D is made, and that has changed a bit over the years, so here is a quick overview. Anti-D is a medicine made from pooled blood. By 'pooled' blood, we mean that donations from a number of people are mixed together to make the Anti-D.

Anti-D is made from the blood of donors who have been sensitised and so are able to produce anti-D antibodies. In a few cases, they became sensitised after accidentally receiving rhesus positive blood (e.g. during pregnancy or a blood transfusion). But many Anti-D donors have been deliberately sensitised, for the sole purpose of being able to donate their blood to make Anti-D. They're very altruistic, lovely people, because they have accepted the small but always present risk that comes from being injected with other people's blood in order to donate blood which will make Anti-D. Not everyone wants to do that; concerns about HIV and potential virus transmission did at one point lead to falls in the number of donors (de Crespigny & Davison 1995). But enough people are volunteering that we haven't run out of Anti-D yet. Some have donated enough blood to make thousands or even tens of thousands of doses. So they're pretty cool people.

Most Anti-D is now made by for-profit biotechnology or pharmaceutical companies, although that hasn't always been the case. In the UK, the company which makes Anti-D used to be state-owned and part of the National Health Service. It is now privately owned. Many Anti-D programmes are still run in conjunction with national blood transfusion services or companies such as Red Cross Australia, even where the Anti-D is manufactured and sold by private companies. In some parts of the world, there is a black market in Anti-D and the blood used to make it. Often, Anti-D needs to be paid for separately by the woman or family, and it's expensive.

Anti-D is also a scarce resource, especially in some areas of the world. Many low- and middle-income countries do not have an effective Anti-D programme (or, in some cases, any Anti-D programme) and/or the Anti-D itself is hard to come by. There have been shortages of Anti-D in high-income countries too. This is one reason why it's important to do research to work out who really is at risk from sensitisation and when. That's so that we can conserve Anti-D for those who really need it. It's one of the reasons that – as I have previously discussed – there is an advantage to offering fetal rhesus group testing to pregnant women, especially when one or both parents are of European descent and thus have a greater chance of having a rhesus negative baby.

One reason for the scarcity is cost, but another is because a donor has to have been sensitised in order to donate blood from which Anti-D can be made. Clearly, anybody who might become pregnant in the future should not be deliberately sensitised. The screening measures and the existence of blood-borne diseases in some populations also mean that a relatively small number of people can donate blood for Anti-D. In some countries, including the USA, Canada, Australia and New Zealand, people who lived in the UK for more than six months between 1980 and 1996 are not able to give blood at all, including for Anti-D, because of the risk of transmission of variant Creutzfeldt-Jakob disease (vCJD), for which there is no screening test. The same precaution does not apply in the UK, because so many residents of the UK fall into that category that, if they were all ineligible to be blood donors, there wouldn't be enough donated blood for those who needed it. On a population level (which is the level at which policy makers need to make decisions), that risk outweighs the risk of vCJD transmission. On the other hand, some people argue that there are ways in which the UK blood donation programme is safer than that of some other countries, and that's because it's voluntary. The reward for donating blood in the UK is half an hour or so in the company of the friendly donation centre staff, followed by a cup of tea and a couple of biscuits. In some countries, such as the USA, people are paid to donate blood, and that can mean that the demographic profile of blood donors is different, with the US programme attracting people who may have lifestyle factors which are more likely to be associated with blood-borne diseases. It's a really complex area which is deeply mired in the different approaches to health care and treatment that exist around the world.

The Anti-D injection – what happens

Many people also have questions about how Anti-D is given, so let's address that next. Anti-D is usually given into a muscle by injection. It used to be injected into the woman's bottom or thigh, but nowadays it's more common to inject it into her arm. This is to ensure that it is given into a muscle and not into fatty tissue. You can always ask if you want it injected into a particular arm, or if you have questions about where it will be injected. Anti-D can also be given into a vein or subcutaneously (under the skin), but this is usually only done when someone has a blood clotting disorder.

Anti-D can be given by midwives, doctors, some nurses and, in some countries, by other health care professionals. The person giving it should check your name, your notes and the details of the injection very carefully. The label from the Anti-D should be placed in your notes or given to you. This is vitally important, because it contains the batch number. Having the batch number ensures that, in the unlikely event of a contamination problem (which I'll discuss in the next section), you will know whether or not it affects you. Always tell the person giving Anti-D to stop if you are unsure or want more information. That goes for any medicine or injection, not just Anti-D.

Anti-D is a thick, yellow substance and it can take a moment or two to inject it fully. A few women say they find it a bit more painful than other injections, but many say that it didn't feel any different. As with all injections, it can sting a bit when the needle goes in, and a few people find that the injection site (for instance their arm or leg) is tingly or numb afterwards.

Because Anti-D is a medicine made from blood, and a very small number of people have an allergic reaction to it, you may be asked to remain in the clinic, surgery or hospital for about twenty minutes after you have it. This ensures that, if you do have a severe adverse reaction, a health professional will be nearby to give you any emergency treatment necessary. The same precaution is taken after giving any blood product. Some midwives and doctors will give the injection at the beginning of your appointment so that you won't have to wait around afterwards. Whether or not you are asked to wait, always tell someone if you feel unwell after having Anti-D.

Common and rare side effects of Anti-D

There are four key types of side effects listed by the Anti-D manufacturers. The first and most common side effect of Anti-D is an injection site reaction (and these are also common after some other types of injections too). These include local inflammation at the injection site, swelling, warmth, redness and soreness. Such reactions are short-lived and don't usually cause problems other than a few days of discomfort.

The second type of side effect is that between one in ten and one in three women have systemic reactions to Anti-D, and these include chills, fever, skin rashes and/or aches (Drugs.com 2020a). I have known several women who suffered an irritating (and sometimes very itchy) body rash after having Anti-D. In more than one case where the Anti-D was given after birth, this hampered breastfeeding and made the first few days of motherhood difficult. We don't have good estimates of the frequency of this type of reaction; it's certainly not common, but it does occasionally happen. This type of reaction can also sometimes happen after someone receives a blood transfusion or another type of medicine made from blood.

The third type of side effect is rare but serious. A severe and immediate reaction is possible with any medicine. But severe reactions, which can include hyper-sensitivity, anaphylaxis or shock, are a bit more likely with blood products and medicines made from blood. This is why women who receive Anti-D may be asked to remain in the clinic or waiting area for twenty minutes or so after it is given. It means that skilled, professional help will be at hand if they need treatment. As far as evidence goes, there have been cases of anaphylactic reactions after Anti-D (Rutkowski & Nasser 2014), but these are rare and generally easily treated. I haven't found any reports of any fatal reactions to Anti-D.

This third category of side effects is the reason why, in many areas of the world, Anti-D can only be given in a hospital or medical clinic and not someone's home. There are two reasons for this. One is because of this chance of a serious allergic reaction that I just described. The second reason is that, in many areas of the world, all blood products and medicines made from blood need to be checked by two registered health professionals. This is to ensure that the right medicine is given to the right person in the right dosage at the right time. This can be really frustrating for those who have a home birth and who wish to have Anti-D but don't want to go to a hospital to have it. If you are told that you will not be able to have Anti-D at home, you can ask about whether other options are available. It may be possible to have Anti-D at a local community clinic, GP surgery or birth centre rather than going to a large hospital. If you think this may affect you, it is a good idea to ask about the options early, so you have time to explore what is available and what will work for you.

The fourth category of possible side effects listed by the manufacturers is that of blood-borne infections. This is a complex issue, so I will look at that separately.

Anti-D and blood-borne infection

Anti-D is a blood product, and as such has the potential to carry infections. The risks of Anti-D are compounded by the fact that the blood used to make the product is pooled, so blood from one infected donor may end up in several hundred doses of the product. Any product made from human blood carries a risk of transmitting infectious agents, which include viruses and the variant Creutzfeldt-Jakob disease (vCJD).

Sadly, many cases of virus transmission occurred in the early years of Anti-D manufacture. In the late 1970s, several thousand women in Ireland contracted hepatitis C from contaminated Anti-D (Meisel *et al* 1995, Reilley & Lawlor 1999, Kenny-Walsh 1999). Hepatitis B was also transmitted through Anti-D manufactured in the German Democratic Republic (Kirchebner *et al* 1994, Schochow & Steger 2020). The virus transmission issue is not unique to Anti-D. The Irish Blood Transfusion Board conducted a tribunal of enquiry into the cases, and found '*many other transmission episodes of hepatitis C virus by immunoglobulin preparations*' (Yap 1997). Anti-D is, however, the only immunoglobulin-based medicine that is routinely offered to childbearing women.

The Irish contamination originated from just one donor but, because of the way Anti-D is manufactured, it affected several batches of the product (Kenny-Walsh 1999). This is the downside of it being made from pooled blood. A later study followed up 682 women who had been infected with hepatitis C from Anti-D given between 1977 and 1979 (Garvey *et al* 2017). The researchers looked at the women's health status in 2013, some 35 years after they had been infected. The women's median age at the time of infection was 28 years, and they ranged from 17-44 years of age. So when the data were gathered for the later analysis, their median age was 63, with the youngest (at that point) being 52 and the eldest 79. The researchers learned that, by the end of 2013, 19% of the chronically infected women had developed cirrhosis, 2% had liver cancer, and 5% had already died from liver-related diseases. At the end of 2013, 321 (86%) of the chronically infected patients remained alive, 247 (77%) of whom were still chronically infected (Garvey *et al* 2017).

In 1989, the HIV virus was also found to have been transmitted in a batch of Anti-D made in India (Malviya *et al* 1989, Dumasia *et al* 1989). Since it became understood that the HIV virus could be transmitted in plasma, routine screening of blood products had been undertaken in most countries. The UK had implemented such screening in 1985 (Hoffbrand *et al* 1999). However, there was (and continues to be) some variation in the standards and screening measures used in different countries.

The issue of viral contamination of blood products and medicines made from blood is a tricky one. The companies who manufacture Anti-D in high-income countries state that known viruses (including hepatitis C and HIV) are now screened for and would be rendered harmless by the purification processes now used. Yet these standards are not universal, and few studies are carried out to test this. Women in low- and middle-income countries do not fare so well. For example, a study of women who had received Anti-D in Baghdad found that *"Anti-HCV, and HCV-RNA seroprevalence were significantly higher (17.1, 35.5%) among women [who had been given] Anti-D..."* (Al-Kubaisy *et al* 2018). These are both markers in the blood which show that somebody has been infected with the hepatitis C virus.

Al-Kubaisy *et al* (2018) also found that the likelihood of someone having been infected with hepatitis C was increased if they had been given more doses of Anti-D. This may sound like it is so obvious that it doesn't need to be mentioned, but, in the absence of having been able to detect the hepatitis C virus in the Anti-D itself or to go back and check the Anti-D (which by then would have been used up), this acts as further confirmation that Anti-D was likely to have been the source of the infection. Overall, Al-Kubaisy *et al* (2018) showed that women who had received Anti-D were 3.6 times more likely to have a positive test for hepatitis C than women who did not receive Anti-D. I want to point out that this number refers to the relative risk. I often tell people to look beyond relative risk, which can make something sound more dangerous (or safer) than it really is. My advice is to also look for the absolute risk of something, because if something was very rare to begin with, then it being twice as likely doesn't really mean that much. Unfortunately, in this case, we just don't have those figures, so I can't give any more information.

Al-Kubaisy *et al*'s (2018) conclusion was to suggest that women who receive Anti-D in pregnancy or after birth should be given hepatitis C tests to see if they have become infected. That's certainly one way of responding to this issue. A more woman-centred approach would be to give the women good information before they need to make this decision so that they can weigh up the pros and cons and the different risks and decide whether or not they want to have Anti-D and, if so, at what point(s) in their birthing journey. This is, as we will return to later in the book, the difference between taking a population-based approach to decision making (which is how recommendations are made) and an approach which focuses on the individual being able to weigh up all of the information and make the decision that is right for them.

It's clear that we could be doing more to help low- and middle-income countries. Most high-income countries have virus screening measures in place which work effectively. Where this is happening, we can be confident that donated blood is being screened for those viruses and infective agents that we know about and have effective means to eradicate. We can (and many Anti-D manufacturers do, though the standards vary a bit between countries) develop means of treating Anti-D and blood products to kill unwanted agents. The concern in high-income countries these days relates to the presence of as yet unknown viruses. As those who have lived through 2020 are now aware, new viruses do appear from time to time. It can take a while for us to learn about them, determine if they are transmissible by blood transfusion and develop the means to treat, vaccinate against and/or eradicate them. This is illustrated by a quote from the June 2020 issue of Transfusion:

"A number of published studies report that the RNA of SARS-CoV-2, the virus causing pandemic COVID-19, is detected in the blood, plasma, or serum of infected people. Unsurprisingly, some of these reports include RNA detection in blood donors. This gives rise to the obvious question: Is SARS-CoV-2 a transfusion-transmitted infection (TTI)? If it is, does it cause a transfusion-transmitted disease (TTD)? We do not know; we think it is unlikely, but we have not proven the negative." (Katz 2020: 1111).

Anti-D researchers and manufacturers continue to develop means of testing and treating as the world tackles new and emerging agents such as Zika and the SARS-CoV-2 virus. But the risk of infection, however low, can't be completely eradicated. Nature, as we were reminded in 2020, isn't predictable or controllable. Again, that applies to any blood product, not just Anti-D.

Finally, I have noted that much of the Anti-D given in high-income countries is made in collaboration with national blood transfusion organisations. This is the case in the UK, many Western European countries, Australia, New Zealand and Canada. In some other areas of the world, including the USA, Central and South America and parts of Africa and Asia, some Anti-D is made by private companies and/or can be bought by those in private practice. Instances of inadequately filled syringes and other problems have been recorded (Moise 2002) and quality standards may be less stringent. Don't hesitate to ask about the source of Anti-D if you have concerns.

Midwives' and parents' concerns

I want to mention a couple of other issues relating to side effects which are often discussed amongst concerned parents, midwives and other birth workers. In the past, concerns were raised because some forms of Anti-D contained a mercury-based preservative called thiomersal (which is also known as thimerosal). Some women declined Anti-D or limited their exposure to it because of concerns about potential toxicity and neurological effects. Thiomersal is no longer used in the manufacture of any of the preparations of Anti-D that I am familiar with. But you always have the right to ask for details of any medicine that you are offered and these days it is simple to look up product information on the internet.

A number of people, including several midwives, have expressed concern about the possibility of longer-term effects of Anti-D, but these have never been adequately researched. Ina May Gaskin (1989), an American midwife, was one of the first to raise concerns about the effects of Anti-D. She noticed similarities between the issues in this area and the work of Durandy *et al* (1981), who studied the effects of the administration of gamma globulin to children between the ages of four and ten years. While the children did not show negative effects of this immediately, the researchers found that their immune systems were compromised for up to five months after receiving the gamma globulin. Over the past twenty or so years, I have met and heard from a significant number of women who have felt that they experienced a longer-term reaction after having Anti-D, which rendered them more susceptible to viruses and infections. It is likely that I have heard about these cases because of my work on Anti-D, but that does not negate these women's experiences.

No research has been undertaken to look at potential long term effects of Anti-D. This is despite women, midwives and doctors calling for more research for many years (Hensleigh 1983, Harmon 1987, Gaskin 1989, Romm 1999, Wickham 2001). Concerns have also been expressed about the effect that Anti-D given in pregnancy might have on the unborn baby, and I will look at this further in the next chapter. Midwives also note that they and their colleagues are often not supported to offer balanced information about Anti-D. Some have questioned the language of the guidelines and recommendations, which are often written in a patriarchal tone as well as not being based on robust evidence of benefit (Wickham 2001, Harkness 2015, Harkness *et al* 2016).

These other side effects of Anti-D would not be easy to research. It would be difficult to separate out the effects of Anti-D from the effects of being pregnant, giving birth and potentially having other drugs and interventions in association with that. But the lack of evidence for this stems from a lack of research, which means we just don't know whether this is more likely in those who have had Anti-D or something that is equally likely to be experienced by women who haven't had Anti-D.

A final side effect of Anti-D to be aware of (although it won't hurt you physically) is that having Anti-D can mean that, if your blood is then tested, you may be found to have anti-D antibodies in your blood. That doesn't necessarily mean you are sensitised. The antibodies may be from the manufactured Anti-D and they will not remain in your blood for long. But if you received Anti-D and want to find out if you have become sensitised, it is not possible to know right away. It is not possible to tell whether any antibodies that show up are from your own body or from the manufactured Anti-D. But this is, for most people, more of an annoyance that needs to be talked through with your care provider if you end up facing such a decision rather than a reason to avoid having Anti-D. It's just something to be aware of.

As with any medicine, the key is to weigh up the risks of the side effects against the benefits of Anti-D. All of the side effects that I have mentioned so far relate to the woman into whose body the Anti-D is injected. When we're giving Anti-D after birth, that's the only person we need consider. When Anti-D is given in pregnancy, however, there is also the question of the effects on the unborn baby. I will look at this question in more depth in the next chapter, when I will look at the evidence relating to the use of Anti-D in pregnancy as part of a wider conversation about the evidence that we can draw on when considering the different aspects of Anti-D.

Making decisions about Anti-D

If you read any information leaflet about Anti-D, it will tell you that Anti-D is very effective at preventing sensitisation and thus rhesus disease in future babies. I'll explain more about that in the next chapter. But whether or not a medicine is effective is only one of the things that people need to consider when making decisions about their health care. That's because all drugs, treatments and interventions have downsides as well as benefits. It's also because, while recommendations are made on a population level (that is, policymakers decide what will be offered across the board, to everyone in a particular situation), we are all individuals.

We're all different. We have different priorities, health histories, backgrounds and contexts, mindsets, family and living situations, and all of these things can affect how something might affect us and what we might want.

I have developed an acronym for people wanting to think about different aspects of a preventative intervention. My acronym, which you may have come across in my other books (Wickham 2017, 2018a) is PIEDAY. Each letter stands for a key bit of information about preventative interventions that you might be offered. Here's a quick overview of the different elements of my PIEDAY acronym in relation to Anti-D, which I want to offer before I detail the evidence in chapter three.

1. What is the **problem**? That is, what problem are we trying to prevent, and how serious is the problem? In the case of Anti-D, we're trying to prevent rhesus negative women becoming sensitised to the anti-D antigen. This is so that any future rhesus positive babies they become pregnant with are not in danger from rhesus disease. I explained rhesus disease and its prevalence in chapter one, but I'll add more on the history of that in chapter three, as it sets the scene for the story of how the evidence came about.

2. What is the **incidence**? We can ask how likely it is that a woman will become sensitised without prophylaxis. I'll discuss that question in the next chapter as well.

3. How **effective** is prophylaxis? We need to ask how well Anti-D (or any preventative measure) works to prevent a problem. I've already mentioned that Anti-D is very effective. But there are different ways of looking at and measuring effectiveness and this is a key issue when it comes to Anti-D, so I'll explore this further in chapter three.

4. What are the **downsides**? Are there risks of the treatment, and how common are they? I looked at the side effects of Anti-D for women earlier in this chapter, so I won't revisit those, but I will look at safety for the unborn baby, and explore some of the wider issues in chapters three and four.

5. Are there **alternatives** to the prophylactic medicine or treatment? Well there are no alternative preventative medicines that do the same job as Anti-D. But in a wider sense, your options include declining Anti-D or having it in some situations but not others. In chapter three, I'll discuss how many women might become sensitised without Anti-D. I will also look at whether there are things one can do to reduce the likelihood of a fetomaternal transfusion. I will come back to that question in chapter four as well. However, because research has focused on Anti-D, the only knowledge we have of possible alternatives is based on theory, experience and anecdote. It's interesting to ponder, but many people would not consider it valid as a basis for making decisions, especially about something that can have such long-term consequences.

6. Finally, I suggest that people need to consider what is right for **you**, as an individual or family. The first part of this involves considering whether there are things about particular people or situations that change any of the population-level information. For instance, if a drug doesn't work as well in people with blue eyes, or if the incidence of the problem is higher in an area. I will touch on that in the next chapter, and there's more on this in chapter four. In theory, we can then identify subsets (or smaller groups) of people who may have less need for Anti-D. Sadly, though, we don't have enough research to be confident in providing advice about whether to have Anti-D or not.

The second part of the 'what's right for you' question involves the way in which it is important to consider one's own health history, family situation, thoughts, beliefs, feelings and ability to cope in different situations, as all of these factors and more can make a difference as to whether a decision or intervention is right in your individual circumstances. I already mentioned (earlier in this chapter) some situations where someone may not want to have Anti-D, for instance if a woman is certain that the baby she is pregnant with will be her last. But, when it comes to Anti-D, the question, 'what's right for you' can also help you think about the fact that Anti-D isn't just offered once. It is offered in several different situations throughout pregnancy and after birth, and some people decide to have it in some situations and not others. That's because the evidence is a bit different for the different situations and indications. In the next chapter, I will explain that more fully.

3. Anti-D: the story of the evidence

In this chapter, I will look in detail at the evidence relating to Anti-D. People who want to weigh up the pros and cons of Anti-D in different situations and make an informed decision face a real problem in this area. The problem is that there is a real lack of robust evidence which could help answer some of the key questions. The reason for this lack of evidence can be seen clearly if we look at the history of how the evidence, knowledge and recommendations on this topic came about. So I'm going discuss the research relating to Anti-D and how this came to be offered in different situations in chronological order, as this illustrates the problems we face today.

A potted history of rhesus disease

The condition of haemolytic disease of the fetus and newborn (which we now know to be a number of related conditions) was discussed by Plato, who lived about two and a half thousand years ago (Bowman 1998). It has been documented since the seventeenth century (Bowman 1998). In fact, in 1609, a French midwife called Louise Borgeois was the first person to write about the condition, which was then known as hydrops fetalis (Kumar & Regan 2005). But it wasn't until 1938 that scientists suggested this might be caused by an immune reaction in the mother to paternal factors carried by the developing baby (Howard el al 1997a). This is perhaps not as surprising as it might at first sound. Let's not forget that doctors were still recommending bloodletting (or removing some blood from a person's body because it was thought that this would make them healthier) just one hundred years before that. In fact, it was 1838 when Dr Henry Clutterbuck, a lecturer in the Royal College of Physicians in London, wrote that, "...blood-letting is a remedy which, when judiciously employed, it is hardly possible to estimate too highly."

Thankfully, things have moved on. The ABO groups were discovered in 1901 (Choate 2018), and our understanding of the importance of blood grew quickly after that. In 1939, Levine and Stetson observed a condition that they described as 'unexpected intragroup agglutination' in a woman who had given birth to a stillborn baby. The woman had been given a transfusion of her husband's blood and, in the process of observing her response, Levine and Stetson (1939) realised that she had been 'immunised' by her baby, who had inherited an antigen from its father (Choate 2018). Levine *et al* (1941) described this as isoimmunisation and, thanks to scientists elsewhere who were working on the same issue from a different angle, the factor was named after rhesus monkeys who were the unconsenting participants in their experiments. These events led to our understanding of how, if a woman became isoimmunised (or sensitised) after one birth, her later babies would sometimes develop HDFN or rhesus disease, as I have already described.

At that time, paediatric care had evolved to the point where some of the babies who experienced severe rhesus disease could be helped. But not all of them. So the next question which faced doctors, scientists and researchers was whether it was possible to prevent maternal sensitisation (Howard *et al* 1997a) and stop the problem from occurring in the first place. Initially, work was carried out to study the nature of the protection that seemed to be offered to women when their blood group differed from that of the baby they were carrying. Research into this situation -- which we call ABO incompatibility between mother and baby -- led to Clarke *et al*'s (1963) suggestion that the administration of intramuscular Anti-D immunoglobulin might clear fetal red cells from the maternal circulation and prevent rhesus isoimmunisation in women.

The original clinical trials

In order to test this theory, a number of studies were done around the world. Nine major clinical trials were conducted between 1967 and 1971 to test the effectiveness of Anti-D. All showed that Anti-D was effective. Almost all of the women in the groups who received Anti-D were protected from sensitisation. As a result of this research finding, Anti-D was manufactured in bulk and the initial recommendation was made that this should be administered to all rhesus negative women who had given birth to a rhesus positive baby. It was also offered to a woman who had given birth to a baby whose rhesus group was undetermined. This sometimes occurred if tests were inconclusive (because this was fifty years ago and science then wasn't what it is today) or in areas where testing wasn't available. This policy has remained largely unchanged to the present day, with more recent research focusing on the specific dose and the addition of other circumstances in which Anti-D should be offered.

It is interesting to look back at these original research studies, which would not be considered robust by today's standards. That doesn't necessarily mean that their results are invalid but I will explain what the issues are, because it helps illustrate the sort of questions we need to ask when evaluating medical research. It is always a good idea to be curious about how knowledge comes about, as research quality varies a lot.

Generally, in order for a trial to be considered unbiased, participants need to be randomly allocated to either the intervention group (those who received Anti-D) or the control group (those who didn't, or who received a placebo). Well-conducted clinical trials also use an approach called double blinding. This means that neither the participants nor the researchers know who got Anti-D and who got a placebo. Double blinding is often achieved by the use of a placebo pill or injection that is given to those in the control group. A good placebo must resemble the product being tested, but be inert. When randomisation and double blinding are used, the researchers (and those reading the research) can be confident that bias did not enter the trial in this way. Otherwise, the participants' or clinicians' preconceptions of the product being tested may subconsciously influence the results.

Neither of these techniques was used in the majority of the clinical trials for Anti-D. In fact, two of the later groups of researchers (Stenchever *et al* 1970, White *et al* 1970) designed studies in response to what the authors felt were the methodological shortcomings of initial work in this area, namely that randomisation and double blinding had not been used. One of these trials (Stenchever *et al* 1970) was stopped after only 54 women had been entered because Anti-D was made available for all rhesus negative women on the basis of the results of the previous research studies. In some ways this was unfortunate, because the preliminary results of this trial appeared to show that Anti-D was less effective than the results of the other trials had suggested.

The trial by White *et al* (1970) also showed interesting results. A total of 313 women had signed up when it was stopped and the isoimmunisation rate in the control group was the lowest of all of the nine clinical trials. It is, again, impossible to know whether the results of these two trials were a more accurate representation of the effectiveness of Anti-D because randomisation and double blinding was used, or whether (particularly in the case of the Stenchever *et al* (1970) trial) they were less accurate because not enough women had been entered in the trials to make a fair assessment of the effectiveness of Anti-D.

We will never know whether we could have learned more from these discrepancies, but I need to clarify what I mean by that. I am not suggesting that Anti-D is less effective than we think it is. The fact that we see very few cases of rhesus disease these days confirms its effectiveness. But we might have been able to learn helpful things about Anti-D in different women or situations if a bit more research had been carried out. That said, it is usual practice to stop trials in these circumstances, and in modern, technocratic culture it is considered ethical and appropriate to do so. The later trials were stopped because the results of earlier studies showed that Anti-D worked. Continuing to undertake studies would have meant depriving women in the control groups of Anti-D. And by this time, as I noted above, programmes which offered Anti-D after birth were being rolled out in many high-income countries. But just because it is considered ethical to stop a programme of research doesn't mean that the results of that decision aren't really frustrating to those who want to make individualised decisions or to understand the issues more deeply. Early cessation of research has happened (and is still happening) in many other areas of medicine and maternity care, and there are a number of other areas where our knowledge is also lacking as a result of such decisions (Wickham 2017, 2018b, 2019). More on this in chapter four.

It's also important to take a balanced, considered approach to our appraisal of fifty year-old studies and decisions. As someone who teaches research appraisal to midwifery and medical students, could I highlight numerous problems with these studies? Yes. But that's because we have learned a lot in the last few decades. Criticising fifty year old research studies for lack of rigour is a little bit like criticising a film made in the 1960s because its special effects weren't as good as those used today. There is a key difference between studies and films though. Today, we can easily make new films – or re-make old ones – using new technologies and special effects. When it comes to medical research, we generally can't go back and redo studies. That's because it is considered unethical to randomise women into intervention and control groups and thus deprive those in the control groups of Anti-D.

This leaves us with quite a dilemma and, while I will come back to this in depth in chapter four, I think it is important to outline it here, so that you can bear it in mind as you read some of the information in this chapter. The dilemma is that there are some really tantalising questions left in this area, but we are going to struggle to get the answers to them, at least as long as we work within the current framework of western medicine and its approach to research.

Most people aren't concerned with that dilemma. Most people focus on and celebrate the fact that the studies showed that Anti-D was effective. And although I do want to look all around the issues and give you every side of the picture in this book, I also want to keep acknowledging that Anti-D sits at the centre of an incredible success story. In a relatively short time, clinicians and researchers identified the source of a problem, suggested a solution, undertook research to see if their solution worked, determined that it did and then worked with multiple agencies to put together a programme that protected rhesus negative women's future babies. That's brilliant, and those working on this deserve all the accolades and prizes that they received as a result.

The effectiveness of Anti-D

I mentioned near the beginning of this chapter that it was important to look closely at the question of the effectiveness of Anti-D, which was the first thing that researchers had set out to determine. The initial clinical trials gave us information about the effectiveness of Anti-D, but there are a couple of important caveats. First, the early trials focused only on the situation where rhesus negative women were offered Anti-D after the birth of a rhesus positive baby. We'll come back to the other indications (or situations in which Anti-D is offered, such as during pregnancy) later in this chapter.

Second, the type of effectiveness that I'm talking about in this section is the kind that we look at in trials. We actually use the term 'efficacy' to describe this. Medical researchers use the term 'effectiveness' to look at what happens in the real world, and there's an important difference between research efficacy and real world effectiveness. In the real world, people forget to take pills, either by accident or on purpose (e.g. because they don't like the side effects), and occasionally they are given the wrong dose or another error is made. We now have a number of studies which show that Anti-D isn't always offered to the right people at the right time. Systems, pathways and clinicians fail more often than you might think. And, although we have known that this problem exists for a long time (Tovey 1986, Ghosh & Murphy 1994, Howard *et al* 1997a), we have still not fully solved it and it remains a key piece of the puzzle (Fyfe *et al* 2014, Akers *et al* 2018, 2019, Glazebrook *et al* 2020). I will return to that question later too. For now, I'm going to turn to the efficacy of Anti-D within the ideal setting of a clinical trial. How well does Anti-D work to prevent sensitisation if the right medicine is given to the right person at the right time?

As you now know, the results of the trials that I described above showed that Anti-D is very effective in preventing rhesus D sensitisation. That is, the vast majority of women in the study groups who received Anti-D did not become isoimmunised or go on to develop antibodies to the rhesus antigen. As the Cochrane review on *'anti-D administration after childbirth for preventing Rhesus alloimmunisation'* shows, after 6 months, 10/4756 women in the Anti-D group were sensitised (0.2%) compared to 204/2824 women in the control group, which is 7.2% (Crowther & Middleton 1997). I will also note that the Cochrane reviewers also excluded some of the nine trials because they were of really poor quality, and they also noted significant shortcomings with some of the trials they did include. Their analysis of the quality of the studies included several of the points that I raised above.

The Cochrane reviewers also looked at another question. Analysis of a much smaller group of women suggested that, when the researchers compared sensitisation rates in the women who didn't receive Anti-D at the beginning of their next pregnancy, they were higher; in some cases, up to 15% of women had become sensitised by that point. However, it is difficult to know whether the women whose data were gathered for this later analysis were representative of all the women in the study, or the population as a whole, or whether there is a chance that those who were sensitised were more likely to have data collected at this point. If that occurred, then the rate of sensitisation could appear higher than it really is. Or it could be that the opposite is the case: we just don't know.

We do know that, in some of the studies, about one in ten of the women were 'lost to follow up', which means we don't know what happened to them. Given the numbers that are involved here, that's a significant amount of lost data. Were those women lost to follow up because they didn't have a problem in their next pregnancy, which means the inclusion of their data would have brought the sensitisation rate down? Were the data lost because the women and their families moved to a different area? Or maybe they just didn't have another baby? It's frustrating, because there's a big difference between 7.2% and 15%, and there are plenty of people who wish we had better data on this aspect of the studies. Again, we can't go back and repeat this research without depriving some women of Anti-D, and that is deemed unethical.

But let's not forget that, from one perspective, the findings about the effectiveness of Anti-D are really helpful. They are especially helpful if you are a policy maker who wants to offer standardised maternity care which sets out what each woman should be offered. If you can ensure that everyone who works for your organisation offers Anti-D to the right people at the right time, these trials confirm that postnatal Anti-D can be an effective intervention when given on a population basis.

Where this approach is taken, and, as far as our understanding about the effectiveness of Anti-D is concerned, some of the quality issues relating to the research trials don't really matter. We know that giving Anti-D is considerably more effective than doing nothing. If we want the answers to other questions, though, the lack of information and clarity does (again) pose us a bit of a problem.

The unanswered questions

I have already noted that the population-level approach leaves rather frustrating gaps. This became really apparent to me when women first began to ask me questions about this area. Questions like:

If I don't have the postnatal Anti-D, what are the chances that I will become sensitised?

If I decline Anti-D, what's the chance that a future baby will have a problem? And what's the chance that they will have a serious or life-threatening problem?

Is the risk of sensitisation/rhesus disease really high if I don't have Anti-D, or is it quite low but one of those situations where Anti-D is given to everyone 'just in case'?

Those were really good questions. It's important to differentiate questions about sensitisation from questions about rhesus disease, though, for two reasons. One, if later babies are rhesus negative then they aren't at risk from rhesus disease anyway. Two, it's not inevitable that sensitisation leads to severe rhesus disease; some affected babies have a mild form. And, thanks to advances in neonatal care, even the most severely affected babies have a high chance of survival nowadays. In fact, the second question is incredibly hard to answer in a specific way, but my work in the library twenty years ago did at least enable me to start a conversation about the answer to the first.

I will admit that, back then, I was a little surprised to learn the answer. I had gathered the impression, from obstetricians who taught me about Anti-D and related issues, that sensitisation was almost inevitable. But then I dug into the research and found the numbers relating to the proportion of women in the control groups who didn't become sensitised, even without Anti-D. In fact, depending on which figures and timeframe you use, the trial data showed that between 85% and 92.8% of rhesus negative women who had given birth to a rhesus positive baby did not become sensitised, even without Anti-D. So the chance of a woman becoming sensitised without Anti-D wasn't as high as I had been led to believe. But it's certainly not a rare event; a one in seven to one in ten chance is significant, and the fact that sensitisation isn't reversible makes this a rather different decision frame than when we are considering other types of preventative treatments such as vitamin K (Wickham 2017) or antibiotics for Group B strep (Wickham 2019). In both of those situations, it's the current baby who may have a problem. In many cases the problem can be treated (although that is also the case with rhesus disease) but, more importantly, declining these preventative treatments poses no risk to future babies. That's not the case with Anti-D.

What is really unhelpful is that the Anti-D trials weren't able to tell us anything about who is likely to be affected without the medicine or intervention. It could be useful to know, for example, whether there were factors that make it more or less likely that a particular woman could become sensitised. But that's not what those trials looked for. The researchers weren't looking at whether Anti-D was necessary for individual women, or what factors might mitigate the chance of sensitisation. That's not a criticism of the research or the researchers; what they achieved was amazing in the time and context in which they achieved it. It's more of a commentary on the implications of our approach to health care, which focuses on populations and not on individuals.

The trials leave us with some tantalising questions which we have no way of answering. Twenty years on from when I first pointed these things out (Wickham 2001), no other research has considered why most rhesus negative women who give birth to a rhesus positive baby remain unaffected, while a proportion would become sensitised without Anti-D. It is impossible to know from the research findings that we have whether sensitisation might be predictable. We don't know whether protection might be conferred by some pre-existing condition or whether it could be due to differences in care. We have no idea whether different people react differently when it comes to antibody production following exposure to the rhesus antigen. Again, as in so many other areas of maternity care, the focus is always on population-level interventions rather than taking a more individualised approach. And it is now extremely difficult to carry out other kinds of research to explore such areas more deeply, although many women and families want this kind of information.

Despite their limitations, the trials had answered the question that they had sent out to answer: does it work? But so many other questions went unanswered. I will come back to these wider questions later in the book. For now, I want to return to the conversation about the history of Anti-D and the evidence relating to this.

Fifty years of change

Postnatal Anti-D has been offered (at least in high-income countries; the situation varies in middle- and low- income countries) to all rhesus negative women who have given birth to rhesus positive babies since the early 1970s. And it has been very effective, in that the incidence of rhesus disease has been vastly reduced.

It's important to note, though, that the world has seen many other changes in those fifty years. This is a point made by Bennebrock Gravenhorst (1989), who noted that, while the postnatal Anti-D programme was immensely helpful, factors other than the use of Anti-D have also been involved in the decline of rhesus disease. One of these factors is the trend towards smaller families. Before Anti-D was offered to women, rhesus disease often did not manifest until the third or fourth child (Howard *et al* 1997b). As I mentioned in chapter one, improved maternal and neonatal care has also led to a reduction of morbidity (illness) and mortality (death) from rhesus disease. But it can still be a significant problem for those families that are affected, which is why the Anti-D programme has expanded since those original clinical trials.

Anti-D and potentially sensitising events

While the original clinical trials primarily considered the effectiveness of Anti-D given following the birth of a rhesus positive baby, clinicians and researchers were aware that there were other situations where the administration of Anti-D may be appropriate. Over the next decade or so, many countries began to add to the list of situations in which Anti-D should be offered. I'm going to detail how this occurred in the UK, but many other high-income countries followed a similar path. In a nutshell, clinicians decided that Anti-D should be offered for a range of potentially sensitising events.

The initial (1969) UK recommendations were updated by the Standing Medical Advisory Committee in 1976. By that point, these now included the suggestion that a dose of Anti-D should also be offered to rhesus negative women following any miscarriage or abortion after 12 weeks of pregnancy.

This recommendation remains in place today. The 12 week timeframe is significant because there is a general consensus that the chance of sensitisation before 12 weeks of pregnancy is extremely low, with UK guidance now noting that:

"In cases of spontaneous complete miscarriage confirmed by scan where the uterus is not instrumented, or where mild painless vaginal (PV) bleeding occurs before 12 weeks, prophylactic anti-D immunoglobulin is not necessary because the risk of FMH [feto maternal haemorrhage] and hence maternal exposure to the D antigen is negligible." (Qureshi *et al* 2014).

However, if a woman has had surgery, if bleeding is heavier, if the pregnancy is close to 12 weeks and/or if there is doubt about the dates, Anti-D may be offered. A smaller dose may be offered because of the relative size of the baby. In some countries, such as Australia, Anti-D is offered after the loss of a baby at any gestation (RANZCOG 2019).

This recommendation is not based on robust evidence. As Cochrane reviewers have noted (Karanth *et al* 2013), two small studies were carried out in the 1970s in an attempt to consider this question. One (Keith & Bozorgi 1977) wasn't considered robust enough to include in the Cochrane review. The other (Visscher & Visscher 1972) involved just 48 women who had experienced miscarriage, and the study *"...failed to show any difference in maternal sensitisation or development of Rh alloimmunisation in the subsequent pregnancies."* (Karanth *et al* 2013). Nonetheless, the offer of Anti-D is made in these situations, despite the fact that, *"There are insufficient data available to evaluate the practice of anti-D administration in an unsensitised Rh-negative mother after spontaneous miscarriage."* This is because, as in so many areas, it is felt that it is better to err on the side of caution. As Anti-D is effective after birth, it seemed reasonable to think that it is effective after miscarriage or abortion. We just (again) don't have any data on how many women would be sensitised without it.

In 1981, the recommendation was added that Anti-D be offered to women who experienced PSEs in pregnancy (Standing Medical Advisory Committee 1981). Such events include accidental occurrences (such as abdominal trauma and vaginal bleeding) and medical interventions. The list of PSEs for which Anti-D is offered in the UK can be found in chapter one. I don't have space to include the list for every country but most can be found online by searching 'Anti-D guidelines' (or recommendations) and the name of a country.

As with the offering of Anti-D after miscarriage and abortion at or after 12 weeks of pregnancy, the PSE-related Anti-D recommendations aren't based on robust evidence. There is no Cochrane review of this area and the list of PSEs has emerged from consensus conversations. The most up-to-date UK guidance on Anti-D acknowledges that none of the evidence is of high quality (Qureshi *et al* 2014). This isn't as unusual in maternity care as one might think. Prusova *et al* (2014) analysed the guidelines and recommendations put out by the Royal College of Obstetricians and Gynaecologists (RCOG) and found that only 9-12% of these are based on what is considered to be best quality (Grade A) evidence. Around 40% are based on 'recommended best practice,' or 'expert opinion.' All of the recommendations in the UK guideline on Anti-D are acknowledged to be based on moderate (Grade B) or low (Grade C) quality evidence (Qureshi *et al* 2014).

A lot of what happens in maternity care both in general and in relation to Anti-D is based on expert opinion. However, the definition of expert in this situation is rather narrow. Conversations about Anti-D guidelines have rarely included maternity service users and only very occasionally involved a midwife. In fact, as I will explain in the next section, the key decisions in this area have been made by working groups of obstetricians and haematologists with a special interest in rhesus disease, without reference to anyone else who might have an interest in the area (Robson *et al* 1998).

Giving birth and experiencing PSEs in pregnancy are not the only situations in which Anti-D is offered nowadays. It is also now offered as a routine preventative measure during pregnancy, and this is perhaps the most controversial aspect of the Anti-D programme.

The advent of routine antenatal Anti-D

All of the recommendations that we have discussed so far relate to situations where there is a specific reason to be concerned that a sensitising event may have occurred. We don't have robust evidence to support the idea of offering Anti-D after a PSE in pregnancy, but it's not difficult to understand the reasoning around why this is offered. It seems plausible that fetomaternal transfusion may occur if trauma or blood loss occurs. And, as fetomaternal transfusion may lead to sensitisation, there is good reason to offer Anti-D. It is then up to the individual woman to decide whether or not she wants to have this or not.

The conversation surrounding the routine administration of Anti-D during pregnancy began as far back as 1967, with the suggestion that consideration of antenatal administration may reduce the rate of sensitisation (Zipursky & Israels 1967). Bowman & Pollock (1978) followed this up with the specific recommendation that Anti-D should be administered to all rhesus negative women at 28 weeks of pregnancy to prevent sensitisation in pregnancy. The debate continued throughout the 1980s, and British researchers were divided between those who saw routine antenatal Anti-D as a wholly beneficial intervention that would save babies, and those who urged caution for a variety of reasons. These included side effects, financial cost, the scarcity of Anti-D, the fact that we knew very little about potential side effects on unborn babies and also the desire not to give women more of a blood-derived medicine than was necessary.

By the late 1990s, there was growing concern that a small number of women were still becoming sensitised, even though Anti-D was – at least in theory – being offered in all the situations that I have described in this chapter (Robson *et al* 1998, Qureshi *et al* 2014). Some countries, such as Germany (Schlensker & Kruger 1996), began offering routine antenatal Anti-D at this time. A number of reviews of the effectiveness of the existing Anti-D programme in countries such as the UK had highlighted that some women were still becoming sensitised (Tovey 1986, Huggon & Watson 1993, Ghosh & Murphy 1994, Howard *et al* 1997a, ACOG 1999). In some cases, this was found to be due to 'failure of administration,' which means that, in practice, Anti-D wasn't always offered to the right people at the right time. For instance, Tovey (1986) analysed cases of sensitisation that occurred in Yorkshire, England between 1980 and 1983. It was discovered that 36 of these cases were due to failures of administration, and such failures accounted for 22% of the women who became sensitised. Howard *et al*'s (1997) study showed that 39% of the cases of sensitisation found in their study were due to failure of administration. Ghosh and Murphy (1994) looked at Scottish data and discovered many instances where women had no record of Anti-D being offered or administered on their notes, and only 69.6% of women who experienced a PSE in pregnancy were offered Anti-D.

This is where we need to consider the second kind of effectiveness that I described near the beginning of this chapter. We saw from the initial clinical trials that, if Anti-D is given in the right dose to the right person at the right time, it's effective. But the effectiveness of the Anti-D programme as a whole is another issue, so let's take a closer look at that.

In order for a programme of intervention to be effective, a lot of things need to work well and together. First, the Anti-D programme involves a lot of professionals working in a lot of areas. There are the midwives working directly with women and families in their homes and on hospital wards. They offer information, take blood, give Anti-D and make records in women's notes. Whether a woman gives birth in hospital or at home, quite a few people are involved in getting Anti-D prescribed, transported and given. In a hospital, once the midwife has taken the blood, the ward clerk will likely contact the hospital porters, who take the blood to the laboratory. When women give birth at home, the midwife may take the blood to a laboratory or collection point themselves. In the laboratory, there are medical laboratory scientists who test the blood. Haematologists may advise in complex situations, for instance where the results of a test are unusual or if a woman needs more than the standard dose of Anti-D. Once the scientist has tested the woman's blood, they then issue the Anti-D and it gets transported back to the midwife on the postnatal ward (thank you porters) and then needs to be refrigerated until it is given to the woman. In the case of a home birth, the Anti-D may be sent to the midwife or to the place where it will be given.

I'm not finished yet, though. Because we mustn't forget that pregnant women don't always go to maternity departments if they have an issue in pregnancy. So GPs, practice nurses, people working in accident and emergency departments and other health care professionals need to know about this as well. All of those professionals need to be aware of the need for testing and offering Anti-D, and they need to know how the system works. They need ongoing education, as the guidelines can (and often do) change.

But we're still not quite done! Then there are a lot of systems which need to work together, including the computer systems, guidelines, maternity records, all the laboratory equipment, testing systems and records and so on. And then there's a time frame in which the woman's blood needs to be taken, tested and the Anti-D issued. I haven't even covered everything that is involved, but this is a broad outline.

I mention all of these things not as an excuse, but as explanation of how the Anti-D programme is really complex. This complexity may be why it is still the case that some women do not get offered the right dose of Anti-D at the right time and we see 'failure of administration.' We know from several studies that cases of sensitisation as the result of Anti-D not being offered to the right person and in the right dosage at the right time occur around the world and to this day (ACOG 1999, Morrison 2000, Rowley *et al* 2013, Akers *et al* 2019, Visser *et al* 2019, Glazebrook *et al* 2020).

But the introduction of routine antenatal Anti-D involved another important idea. There was also concern that, even if Anti-D was always offered to the right people at the right time in the right dose, a few women would still become sensitised. The thinking was that a few women may experience a PSE during pregnancy without realising. This came to be called 'silent sensitisation' and I will return to discuss this in more depth later in this chapter. I want to mention first that, again, this issue was discussed in a series of meetings that involved doctors, pharmaceutical company representatives and scientists. Few midwives were involved (and certainly none who had concerns about the programme) and, to my knowledge, not a single rhesus negative woman or lay representative was invited. These conversations led to most high-income countries adopting the recommendation that rhesus negative women should be routinely offered prophylactic Anti-D during pregnancy. These countries included the UK, the USA, Australia, New Zealand, Canada and most European countries.

Perhaps because of the controversy over the evidence in this area, there is quite a bit of variation between countries regarding the timing and dosage of routine antenatal Anti-D regimes. For example, Sperling *et al* (2018) compared national recommendations on prevention of sensitisation published by the organisations who formulate guidelines for use in the UK, the USA, Canada and Australia/New Zealand, and they concluded that:

> *"Variation exists in recommendations on the timing and need for consent prior to routine antenatal anti-D immune globulin administration, prophylaxis for unique circumstances (e.g., threatened abortion < 12 weeks, complete molar pregnancy), and the use of cell-free fetal DNA testing for fetal RhD genotype."* (Sperling *et al* 2018).

In my experience, the offer of routine antenatal Anti-D is the element of the Anti-D programme that women and families are most likely to question. A few women do decline Anti-D after birth, but most do not. A few accept Anti-D after birth but will carefully consider whether they want it after a PSE (often out of concern for their unborn baby, whom it will not benefit). The vast majority of women decide to have Anti-D in both of these situations. But more question whether they want to have it as a routine preventative measure, and this is the element of the programme that is most often declined. Let's look at the evidence, as that shows why routine antenatal Anti-D is contentious.

The case for antenatal Anti-D

As I mentioned above, the authors of some of the studies which highlighted 'failure of administration' also argued that, even if Anti-D was always offered to the right person at the right time in the right doses, some women would become sensitised. Hughes *et al* (1994) undertook research in Scotland, for example, and looked retrospectively at 80 babies with rhesus disease who had been born between 1985 and 1990. They felt that they had adequate data to determine the cause of sensitisation in 70 of these pregnancies, and it was found that seven cases were due to sensitisation before 1970 (in other words, before Anti-D was available). Another ten cases of sensitisation could be attributed to clinicians' failure to implement the current programme; that is, they didn't follow the guidelines correctly so some women weren't offered Anti-D that they should have been offered. The other 53 cases were attributed to the failure of the current guidelines to protect against sensitisation. In other words, even if the guidelines were followed to the letter, 53 women would still have been sensitised. Hughes *et al* (1994) argued that routine antenatal administration would have prevented many of these women from being sensitised. The following year, another research team who looked at data from Yorkshire (McSweeney *et al* 1998) came to the same conclusion: professional failure *was* an issue, but there was still a case for offering routine antenatal Anti-D.

Another argument for routine antenatal Anti-D came from a different kind of study in Derbyshire, England. This was one of the first areas of the UK in which women having their first baby were routinely offered two doses of Anti-D during pregnancy and Mayne *et al* (1997) assessed the effectiveness of this intervention. They showed a fall in the mean overall sensitisation rate from 1.12% in 1988-1991 (before the onset of the antenatal programme) to 0.28% in 1993-1995. They also noted that one of the benefits of the programme was an increase in requests from women for Anti-D in response to PSEs in pregnancy. While the study authors suggest that this increase was probably the result of heightened awareness, they do not offer any insight into what difference this alone might have made to the sensitisation rates. It would be really interesting to have more information about this. Because, while informing women may not have reduced sensitisation rates by the same amount that routine antenatal Anti-D did, it might have ensured that more of the women who experienced PSEs knew about the issues and asked for Anti-D. It probably goes without saying, but if the person who is receiving the medicine takes some of the responsibility for ensuring that they get it, it's more likely to be given.

It is worth knowing a bit about the pros and cons of the data that these studies gathered. They were retrospective, so the researchers looked back on events that had already occurred. What they didn't do (and we will come back to this) was to set up a prospective trial where they measured the effectiveness of additional routine antenatal Anti-D (in those women who didn't mind being randomised into a study) on top of the current programme. Instead, they gathered data from women's notes. We know from long experience that medical records are not a reliable source of data. With the best will in the world, people sometimes write in the wrong notes, or forget to note something down and, when these notes are used to collect data for a study, these errors and omissions can lead to incorrect or misleading results.

It may be helpful to have an example here to illustrate that idea. Let's imagine that Helen had a minor car accident, but didn't think to tell her midwife. Or maybe she hadn't been told that it would be important to report such things and to seek midwifery advice if anything like that happened. Helen had an antenatal check a couple of days later, but the midwife didn't ask about PSEs, so nothing was written in Helen's notes. The midwife didn't write down that she didn't ask Helen – and why would she?! We only write down what we actually do and say. No-one documents that they forgot to do something or that they didn't ask a question. Especially as those who forget things often do so because they are really busy and being asked to do more than is reasonable.

When the researchers come along a few months later, they gather up the medical records of women who have been sensitised, and this includes Helen. They see that Helen – who is now sensitised – has nothing written in her notes about any PSE, and no offer of Anti-D, so they decide that this was a case of silent sensitisation. The sensitisation isn't attributed to the failure of the current Anti-D programme, even though that was actually the cause in this case.

We can see from this example that it's possible that there was (and very likely still is) even more professional failure than the researchers found. Proponents of routine antenatal Anti-D would say that this doesn't matter; the real issue is that routine antenatal Anti-D might have protected Helen. And yes, it might; I'm not going to argue with that. But if Helen had been given information, she could have sought help and asked about Anti-D herself. If her midwife had asked about possible PSEs at every visit, she might have picked up that there was a need to offer Anti-D. But let's return to look more closely at this idea of 'silent sensitisation,' because this is a key question here.

The question of silent sensitisation

The case for offering routine antenatal Anti-D is based on the idea that a small number of women experience so-called 'silent' sensitisation. I say 'so-called' only because, as you now know from the previous section, there is a question about whether some cases deemed to be 'silent' might actually not be silent if caregivers were giving more information to rhesus negative women and ensuring that the guidelines around offering Anti-D in response to PSEs were being followed. It's also possible that we could make changes to the design of the systems. I want to be clear that not all of the blame lies in the hands of individual practitioners here.

Many of the studies which were used by policymakers to argue for the implementation of routine antenatal Anti-D – because some women still became sensitised – can also be used to argue against it. That's because there is evidence that many of the women who became sensitised did not actually experience silent sensitisation. They experienced a known PSE which did not result in them being offered Anti-D. The programme failed them. For instance, Ghosh and Murphy's (1994) Scottish study showed that just over 30% of women who had experienced a PSE in pregnancy had not been offered Anti-D. This is one example of a situation where it would have been so useful to have some qualitative research alongside the quantitative (or number-based) studies. If we had interviewed the women who had been sensitised, would we have found that more of them had a PSE that wasn't documented? But, as is so often the case in medical research, the recipients of care weren't asked about their experiences.

I have mentioned that part of the problem occurs outside of maternity care departments, where staff generally know all about Anti-D. Research in accident and emergency (A&E) departments (Huggon & Watson 1993) found that only eight out of the 29 women who arrived following a threatened miscarriage were offered a test to find out their blood group. In other words, 72.5% of the women weren't offered this. None of the (known) rhesus negative women were offered Anti-D. Following this small study, a larger review of UK A&E departments was carried out by Gilling-Smith *et al* (1998). Of the 88 A&E units that dealt with women who experienced bleeding in early pregnancy, only 23% administered Anti-D when it was appropriate. There were other worrying findings. Only 84% of the units could actually obtain Anti-D, while 37% did not have access to Kleihauer testing to determine whether a woman had experienced a larger bleed than would be covered by the standard dose.

Elsewhere, Howard *et al* (1997a) examined the notes of 922 women who gave birth in seven hospitals, and found that only 20% (so one in five) of women who had experienced abdominal trauma had been offered Anti-D. This study also identified problems with some professionals' understanding of the appropriate doses in pregnancy. Both of these failures are likely to lead to an increase in sensitisation, which clearly cannot be attributed to 'silent' events. As a result, Howard *et al* (1997a) suggested that we should evaluate the effect of applying the existing recommendations more carefully before implementing routine antenatal prophylaxis or considering the use of higher doses of Anti-D. This study also reported only 95% adherence to the recommendation to offer postnatal Anti-D. Medical notes relating to women who did not receive Anti-D did not record that women declined this, which leads to the assumption that it was simply overlooked by clinicians.

These studies are rather old now, and they may not reflect the current situation. I mention them here to illustrate the data that were available when the decision to implement routine antenatal Anti-D was made. And also because, now that routine antenatal Anti-D is offered to all rhesus negative women, it is hard to gather more data which might help us look at the question of whether and how often silent sensitisation occurs. We do, however, know from recent studies that there are still failures of administration. Several recent reviews of research have shown the implementation of the Anti-D programme is still suboptimal. That is, Anti-D is not always being offered to the right women in the right dosage at the right time (Akers *et al* 2018, 2019, Fyfe *et al* 2020, Glazebrook *et al* 2020, Tneh *et al* 2020).

This begs the question of to what extent we're routinely giving a medicine in pregnancy to counteract mistakes that are being made in health care systems. Again, it's not always the direct fault of individual professionals, although sometimes it is. Some people argue that care should be more standardised because of this problem. But some of the mistakes derive from the fact that care is standardised rather than individualised, and that professionals are given less time and expected to do more things within it. As Kirkham (2018) explains, the business model used in modern health care is not compatible with midwifery values, and guidelines can restrict thinking.

There were – and there still are – other options. Rather than giving routine antenatal Anti-D because some clinicians fail to offer this to the women that really need it, we could have considered how the current programme might be better implemented. It would also be useful (not least for those individuals who need to make decisions about Anti-D and who are reluctant to have more Anti-D than is genuinely warranted) to establish how many women are sensitised as a result of failure to implement the current guidelines. As I noted in chapter one, some people consider it less than ideal for women to have to take responsibility for this themselves. But I know from long experience that there do exist many women who would rather take this responsibility than have more Anti-D than is necessary, especially in pregnancy.

I will return to discuss some of these issues more widely in chapter four. But first let's turn to the evidence for antenatal Anti-D and consider whether this intervention is supported by the findings of robust randomised controlled trials.

Routine antenatal Anti-D: the randomised trials

To date, there have been only two trials of antenatal Anti-D which were of sufficient quality to be considered for inclusion in the Cochrane review on this (McBain *et al* 2015). The decision to recommend routine antenatal Anti-D was based on other kinds of data and on more 'expert opinion.' I will discuss that further in the next section. The Cochrane reviewers summarised the situation as follows:

"The quantity of available evidence to answer such an important question of policy was disappointingly low and there was a moderate to high risk of bias in the included studies. We included only two studies in this review, with a total of over 4500 women; one trial was quasi-randomised." (McBain *et al* 2015).

In one of the studies (Lee & Rawlinson 1995), women in the treatment group were given two doses of 50µg (250 iu) of

Anti-D at 28 and 34 weeks of pregnancy. There were no statistically significant differences between their outcomes and those of the women in the group who had not received routine antenatal Anti-D. There were significant flaws in study design and some missing information, rendering the study at unclear risk of bias (McBain *et al* 2015). There was no blinding, not enough detail about randomisation to tell whether this was carried out in a robust manner, and nearly a quarter of all of the women (23%) were 'lost to follow up,' which means we do not know what happened in their cases. This is a bit of a recurring theme with Anti-D research.

Researchers in the other study (Huchet *et al* 1987) gave a larger dose of Anti-D (500 iu) at 28 and 34 weeks and showed a clear reduction in the incidence of sensitisation at between 2 and 12 months. But this study was found to be at risk of bias in a number of ways (McBain *et al* 2015). The trial was quasi randomised, which means that women were not randomly assigned to receive Anti-D or no Anti-D, and this means that there was a high risk of selection bias. No placebo was used. Data regarding subsequent pregnancy were not available and there were incomplete outcome data; 1969 women began the study but only 940 were included in the final analysis. While some of the exclusions were justified and/or unavoidable (e.g. because women were rhesus positive), many were not.

McBain *et al* (2015) are fairly clear in their assessment of the evidence in relation to the routine administration of antenatal Anti-D:

"Existing studies do not provide conclusive evidence that the use of anti-D during pregnancy benefits either mother or baby in terms of incidence of Rhesus D alloimmunisation during the pregnancy or postpartum, or the incidence of neonatal morbidity (jaundice) (low to very low quality evidence). However women receiving anti-D may be less likely to register a positive Kleihauer test in pregnancy and at the birth of a Rh-positive infant (low quality evidence). Fewer

women who receive anti-D during pregnancy may have Rhesus D antibodies in a subsequent pregnancy, with benefits for the baby, however this needs to be tested in studies of robust design." (McBain *et al* 2015).

This was also the conclusion of a recent review of the evidence in this area by a team of Canadian researchers who looked at the evidence for Anti-D in relation to PSEs (both in pregnancy and at birth) and routine antenatal administration:

"Serious risk of bias and low to very low certainty of the evidence is found in existing RCTs and comparative observational studies addressing optimal effectiveness of Rh immunoprophylaxis. Guideline development committees should exercise caution when assessing the strength of the recommendations that inform and influence clinical practice in this area." (Hamel *et al* 2020).

The researchers who led the antenatal Anti-D research in Yorkshire offered a tantalising theory, based upon their data, that women may not need routine Anti-D in later pregnancies if they had it in their first:

"Most advocates of antenatal prophylaxis advise giving anti-D immunoglobulin to unsensitised Rh(D)negative mothers in every pregnancy, but our experience suggests that this may not be necessary. Many of the patients in the Yorkshire trial had four or more pregnancies, and ... only one produced anti-D antibody in her second pregnancy, none in the third, and only one in the fourth even though antenatal prophylaxis was given only in the first pregnancy. This emphasises the importance of the mother's immunological response to the first Rh(D) positive stimulus and the advantage of modifying it by giving anti-D immunoglobulin." (Thornton *et al* 1989: 1672).

This finding has never been followed up. But, as is the case with a number of other interventions within maternity care, a lack of robust evidence has not proven to be a barrier to the widespread implementation of routine antenatal Anti-D.

There are as many stories about how the implementation of antenatal Anti-D came about as there are countries which have implemented a programme. In the next section, I will tell the story of how this intervention was implemented in the UK. That's because the UK story is a really good way of illustrating how medical ideas turn into guidelines and become usual practice, even when there isn't robust underpinning evidence to support their value.

The consensus conference

In 1997, a consensus conference was held to determine a national recommendation (for the UK) for the use of antenatal Anti-D administration. The conference was held jointly by the Royal College of Physicians of Edinburgh and the RCOG.

Conference attendants were said to include a *'range of perspectives'* (Urbaniak 1998) but the majority of participants were haematologists or obstetricians. A number of people and groups were not represented. Childbirth organisations and childbearing women were not invited, and at the time there were also concerns about the lack of clinical midwifery representation within the group. It probably goes without saying that no other birth workers or activists were involved either. This seems rather undemocratic, as it is women who receive Anti-D and usually midwives who inform them of the issues and administer it. Midwives are ideally placed to discuss concerns and could have shared details of the issues, questions and concerns that women and families raise. Midwifery regulators tried to raise concerns about the lack of testing of Anti-D for routine use in pregnancy, reiterating that there was no sound evidence to suggest antenatal administration was beneficial (Coombes 1999). They also highlighted the fact that up to 40% of the 100,000 or so women who would receive antenatal Anti-D each year in the UK would be carrying rhesus negative babies, and therefore would have received this unnecessarily. Childbirth and midwifery organisations (RCM 1999) were equally concerned that women should be able to make decisions based on the evidence available, rather than the opinions of a group of people who may have a different ideology from that of the women and families affected.

The conference was co-sponsored by the blood products industry. One paper that defended the conference described those who pointed this fact out as *"cynics"* and claimed that, *"This is unfair criticism. The evidence of scientific effectiveness of routine anti-D prophylaxis is very robust and on that conclusion alone, the practice must be recommended."* (James 1998). Since that time, the writers of the UK guideline on Anti-D (Qureshi *et al* 2014), the Cochrane reviewers (McBain *et al* 2015) and the authors of a recent Canadian review (Hamal *et al* 2020) have all stated that the evidence on which this conclusion was based is of low certainty.

The consensus conference noted that, *"...there is abundant evidence that the recommendations are not being fully applied..."* (Urbaniak 1998). Robson *et al* (1998) reported the consensus conference's estimate that between 2500 and 3000 women need to be given antenatal Anti-D in order to prevent one death from HDFN. Neither this paper nor the proceedings of the consensus conference where it was discussed showed how this figure was calculated, however. Since my own research into this area began, I have had conversations with some of the researchers who were involved in the conference and the related research, and at least three of those I have spoken to believe that the actual number of women who need to be given antenatal Anti-D to prevent one death from HDFN is higher than this. None were willing to let me cite their names in this book. The number of women who need to be given routine antenatal Anti-D in order to save one baby also increases as neonatal care improves. However, the decision of the consensus conference was to offer routine antenatal Anti-

D to all rhesus negative women regardless of concerns and without seeking further views. This recommendation remains in place today.

The different antenatal Anti-D regimes

Regimes of routine antenatal Anti-D administration differ around the world (Sperling *et al* 2018). There are two main regimes in use. One is a two-dose regimen, wherein a dose of 500iu of Anti-D is offered at both 28 and 34 weeks of pregnancy. The other, which appears to be more common nowadays, is a single dose regimen, where a larger dose of 1500iu of Anti-D is offered between 28 and 30 weeks of pregnancy.

The single dose regime may be more cost effective and, because there is only one injection to give, it is more likely to be given in full than the two-dose regime (Pilgrim *et al* 2009, Qureshi *et al* 2014). But some researchers argue that the two-dose regimen is better because small-scale research has found that women who have two doses have more circulating Anti-D in their blood (White *et al* 2019). As a side note, we can't tell from a blood test whether this is just pharmacological Anti-D (from the medicine) or physiological anti-D (produced by the woman's body). But the assumption is that it is Anti-D the medicine). Having more circulating Anti-D is deemed to be better, because it means that there is more Anti-D to clear any fetal blood cells.

Both the single dose and two-dose regimes are in use in the UK. The single dose regime is recommended by the American College of Obstetricians and Gynecologists (ACOG 2017) in the USA, for example, while RANZCOG (2019) recommend the two-dose regime in Australia (where the two-dose study was carried out) and New Zealand but with 625iu, which is the dose that RANZCOG recommend as standard.

Again, I want to stress that these numbers are what is recommended. The dose of Anti-D given in practice may be different from this, usually because of local availability. I explained earlier in the book that, in the UK, for instance, the recommended postnatal dose is at least 500iu, but some units give 500iu and some give 1500iu doses. It's the same with the doses given in pregnancy. If you are considering Anti-D and wish to know what dosage you would be offered in a given situation, I recommend that you ask a local midwife or doctor what is actually available and offered where you are.

The safety of antenatal Anti-D

The question of whether antenatal Anti-D is safe for the growing baby is hotly debated. I will not discuss the side effects of antenatal Anti-D for women again here, because these were covered at the end of chapter two. But when Anti-D is given in pregnancy – either in response to a PSE or as a routine precaution – there is also the unborn baby to consider. We do know that Anti-D given to a woman can cross the placenta (Maayan-Metzger *et al* 2014), but the question of whether it causes problems is difficult to answer.

The safety of medicines for unborn babies is a tricky issue, and there is significant variation in statements about the safety of antenatal Anti-D. For instance, Drugs.com is a trust run by pharmacists which summarises information about medicines and their uses and side effects. It is trusted by many health professionals as a reliable source of data on the side effects of different medicines, and this is its summary of the use of Anti-D in pregnancy:

"This drug should be used during pregnancy only if the benefit outweighs the risk to the fetus. Some formulations are not approved for use during pregnancy. The manufacturer product information should be consulted. Animal studies have not been conducted.

Available evidence does not suggest harm to the fetus or future pregnancies when given to Rho(D) negative women during pregnancy. There are no controlled data in human pregnancy." (Drugs.com 2020b).

This and similar summaries state that we know very little about the potential effects of Anti-D on unborn babies, because little research has been done. When you consult Anti-D product information leaflets, as this summary suggests, you tend to find similarly vague statements because, again, we have no controlled data on this. However, this statement is interpreted differently by different people, companies and countries. Some people will tell you that we have no evidence that Anti-D might have harmful effects on unborn babies. That is true, but it's important to note that this might be because we haven't carried out many studies to look for the evidence; that's what it means when it says (in the quote above) that, *'there are no controlled data in human pregnancy'* (Drugs.com 2020b). Others will tell you that we have no evidence of safety. That is partly true, and I'll return to a discussion of this point below.

Is it significant that some of the companies who make Anti-D state that it has not been approved for use in pregnancy? Well, the issue there is that quite a lot of drugs haven't been approved for use in pregnancy, and that's usually because they haven't been adequately researched. This is all very unhelpful, I know, and I wish I could offer more, but I can't, because the studies just haven't been done.

But when one digs into the conversations about the safety of antenatal Anti-D, there is a somewhat worrying trend towards stating things which aren't exactly true. In the Cochrane review on routine antenatal administration of Anti-D, which is very honest about the poor quality of the evidence in other areas, McBain *et al* (2015) note the potential risk of transmission of blood-borne diseases but also state that:

"Numerous studies have suggested that while small amounts of passive anti-D may cross the placenta, the antenatal administration of anti-D IgG does not have adverse consequences for the fetus (Liumbruno et al 2010)." (McBain *et al* 2015).

When that review first came out, I was interested by the reference to Liumbruno et al (2010). I hadn't seen that paper, and I eagerly went to look at it, hoping that it would give me some evidence with which I could reassure women and families who were continuing to ask me about the safety of antenatal Anti-D. I was rather disappointed by what I found, and I want to share the details of this with you, because this illustrates why it is so valuable and important to dig a bit deeper and not assume that others have the same values as you do when it comes to citing evidence for their claims.

Liumbruno *et al* (2010) cite a number of references for their statement about the safety of antenatal Anti-D, although some of them simply point to each other and a couple of them are forty year old papers written by the same author that did not focus on safety (Bowman & Pollock 1978, Bowman 1978). So it was immediately apparent that the reference to 'numerous' studies in the quote above was perhaps not a fair description of the volume or quality of the data allegedly 'proving' safety. In fact, only three of the citations mentioned by Liumbruno *et al* (2010) and later cited by McBain *et al* (2015) include data relating to safety. These were all published in the 1980s, and I will explain the content of each in turn, so that you can make up your own mind about whether you agree with McBain *et al*'s (2015) assertion.

The first is a paper published in the American Journal of Obstetrics and Gynecology by Hensleigh (1983), who was actually highlighting his own concerns about the safety of antenatal Anti-D. The author began his discussion on safety by noting that:

"An aura of safety for the fetuses of mothers treated with Rho (D) immune globulin (human) during pregnancy has evolved. This is based mainly on several relatively small studies, each limited to evaluation of cord blood hemoglobin, bilirubin, and direct Coombs tests. None of the large clinical trials of antepartum prophylaxis has collected treatment and control data on fetal losses, birth weights, neonatal morbidity or mortality, neonatal immunologic status, or childhood illnesses. This is particularly unfortunate and clearly a departure from the general guidelines for evaluating new uses of medicinal agents when the fetus is exposed." (Hensleigh 1983:753).

So Hensleigh (1983) acknowledges that a few small studies had been carried out, but argues that these weren't robust enough to evaluate safety, and didn't look at the right things. He is saying the very opposite from what people later claim he said. Hensleigh (1983) goes on to note how difficult it is to research the effects of medicines on babies in utero. This is especially tricky when the unborn baby will not itself benefit from the medicine, as with Anti-D. There is a real irony here. Because one reason for our lack of safety data is that western medical ideology deems it more acceptable to expose a baby to a medicine in the course of routine obstetric practice than to carry out research to assess its safety. Furthermore:

"...to undertake a new treatment without insisting on careful evaluation of other potential adverse effects on the fetus and neonate and without careful assessment of the extent of maternal benefit, is a departure from standard evaluation of new treatments that involve fetal exposure. When one predicts benefit to only one in several hundred patients treated, these considerations must be carefully weighed. An argument could be made that the potential risks for the fetus from antepartum Rho (D) immune globulin (human) treatment of the mother are so minimal as to negate the need for careful study of exposed fetuses. However, the principle of caution when one considers usage of drugs in pregnancy is borne out by several studies which illustrate possible mechanisms for fetal risk which could be relevant to antepartum use of Rh0 (D) immune globulin (human)." (Hensleigh 1983: 753).

The potential risks that Hensleigh (1983) goes on to discuss include possible adverse effects on the growing baby's immune system. He cites research by Durandy *et al* (1981) in children who experienced immunologic effects after receiving gamma globulin which does (Hensleigh argues) imply that unborn babies may experience *"...similar or even more profound effects."* (Hensleigh 1983: 753). As others have noted since, he points out that we do not know what the effects of exposing rhesus positive babies to Anti-D will be in the long term. A particularly important question is whether and how female babies might be affected when they are pregnant with rhesus positive babies.

Hensleigh (1983) discusses other theoretical risks which, to my knowledge, have still not been adequately researched. He concludes with the following statement:

"Neither widespread nor selective antepartum use of Rho (D) immune globulin (human) can be recommended because of marginal benefits, great cost, and lack of adequate fetal safety studies. A more rational approach to further reduction of Rh-hemolytic disease of the newborn rests on the perfecting and clinical application of a sensitive screening test that will identify the few Rh-positive (fetal) cells in the blood of the Rh negative gravid patient. By this means, only those mothers who are truly at risk will be subjected to the cost and fetal exposure inherent in antepartum Rho (D) immune globulin (human) treatment." (Hensleigh 1983: 755).

Given this conclusion, it is hard to understand why Hensleigh's (1983) paper, one of a tiny number that honestly acknowledge the lack of data on safety, is cited as a reference to support the safety of antenatal Anti-D for the fetus in utero.

The second citation on the safety of Anti-D in pregnancy is a letter by Tabsh *et al* (1984) which was also published in the American Journal of Obstetrics and Gynecology. They acknowledge earlier research by Miles and Kaback (1979), who, "...*reported possible adverse effects of anti-D immunoglobulin including a higher rate of fetal loss when anti-D immunoglobulin was administered prior to 20 weeks' gestation.*" I should note here that, while Anti-D might be given after a PSE before 20 weeks of pregnancy, routine antenatal prophylaxis is not offered before this time.

In the hope of determining whether Miles and Kaback's (1979) findings were true of other populations, Tabsh *et al* (1984) carried out a retrospective review of the medical records of 300 women who had antenatal Anti-D after amniocentesis. Their outcomes were compared to a control group of rhesus negative women. The conclusion was that:

"*In the present retrospective study, no significant differences were seen in the incidence of pregnancy wastage* [sic, this is a horrid term used to describe the loss of a baby], *intrauterine growth retardation, preterm delivery, mean birth weight, and congenital defects between the group of patients receiving anti-D immunoglobulin and the control group.*"(Tabsh *et al* 1984: 226).

In one sense, this is reassuring. But it is also important to acknowledge that neither Miles and Kaback's (1979) nor Tabsh *et al*'s (1984) research was robust enough for us to be confident of their findings, and I find it surprising that the Cochrane reviewers (McBain *et al* 2015), who have rejected similarly weak studies in their review, have relied on an interesting but not robust paper to support their statement about the 'numerous studies' evidencing the safety of antenatal Anti-D. Tabsh *et al* (1984) themselves conclude that:

"*Further prospective studies need to be performed to confirm the safety of anti-D immunoglobulin administration in the second trimester of pregnancy.*" (Tabsh *et al* 1984: 226).

The third actual paper cited by Liumbruno *et al* (2010), and thus by the Cochrane reviewers, as evidence of the safety of antenatal Anti-D, is a study by Thornton *et al* (1989). This one is also a retrospective study but it is of more robust design, not least because it came a few years later and at a time when our understanding of how to carry out research effectively was growing. The authors have discussed Hensleigh's (1983) concerns about antenatal Anti-D on babies in utero, but let's look first at the details of the study.

Thornton *et al* (1989) studied data from 17 hospitals in West Yorkshire, England, which had already been collected for another research study (Tovey *et al* 1983). Thornton *et al* (1989) compared the outcomes of two different groups of women, by using information recorded in the women's medical records. The first group included rhesus negative women who gave birth to a rhesus positive baby (who was their first baby) after 34 weeks of pregnancy in 1980 or 1981, which was after the introduction of routine antenatal Anti-D. Then, they compared these women with similar women who had given birth in 1978 and 1979, before routine antenatal Anti-D was in use. So the first group had been given two doses of antenatal Anti-D, but the second group hadn't.

The women who had the antenatal Anti-D were less likely to be sensitised, which isn't a great surprise, because we know that Anti-D is effective, but this research was also concerned with safety. The researchers state that:

"We tried to explore further the safety of antenatal prophylaxis. Among the 1640 mothers who had at least one further pregnancy (889 plus 751) we were able to follow up clinically 1152 (616 in group 1 and 536 group 2, 70%). All the information suggested that the cases were representative, and there was no evidence of different obstetric care. Our results showed no evidence that antenatal prophylaxis was detrimental to either mother or infant. In particular, we cannot support the findings of Tabsch [sic] et al of a trend towards increased perinatal mortality and morbidity in infants whose mothers received anti-D immunoglobulin in the

second trimester after amniocentesis. This discrepancy may well be due to our antenatal prophylaxis being given later in pregnancy or the selection of mothers requiring amniocentesis." (Thornton *et al* 1989: 1672).

It's very useful to know that Thornton *et al* (1989) found no evidence of detrimental effects. A few things need to be borne in mind, though. Their study was retrospective, so the data are less reliable than if they had been collected in a prospective trial that had been designed to compare specific outcomes. They used a smaller dose of Anti-D (100iu) than is currently offered in pregnancy (300iu to 1500iu, depending on where you are in the world). And one of the reasons I went into detail about Hensleigh's (1983) concerns earlier in this section was so that I could point out that, while Thornton *et al*'s (1989) conclusion about safety is reassuring in one sense, their research wasn't actually designed to look for the sort of problems that Hensleigh (1983) and previous researchers were concerned about.

Like so much research in obstetrics, the focus in Thornton *et al*'s (1989) study is on short-term, physical outcomes. While it's useful to know that there was no difference in mortality rates, and babies who were exposed to antenatal Anti-D were not more likely to be ill soon after birth, this wasn't the concern. The concern was (and, for some, remains) about whether being exposed to Anti-D in utero may affect a baby's immune system (which might not be seen at birth but may appear a few months or even years later) and/or whether the baby may experience other effects later in life.

There are a few other useful studies, though none have addressed the bigger safety questions in prospective research. For example, one concern about safety has been about what happens when rhesus positive babies are exposed to Anti-D in utero. Maayan-Metzger *et al* (2001) previously found that 20% of babies in this situation had a positive Coombes test, which means that Anti-D was circulating in their blood. The lead researcher also carried out a later study, collecting data (again retrospectively) on 94 babies born prematurely (at between 28 and 34 weeks of pregnancy) after their mothers had received Anti-D. In this study, 11.7% of the babies had a positive Coombes test and the exposed babies had higher bilirubin levels than matched counterparts who had not been exposed to Anti-D. Their bilirubin levels remained higher for three days after birth, but:

"No differences between study and control groups were recorded for hematocrit levels throughout hospitalization, maximal bilirubin level, phototherapy duration and day of initiation or need for blood transfusion." (Maayan-Metzger *et al* 2014: 907).

The researchers concluded that, *"Further prospective studies are needed to confirm these findings in order to support anti-D administration close to preterm birth."* (Maayan-Metzger *et al* 2014: 90).

I have not found any more recent studies on this topic.

Like Hensleigh, I find it interesting to contemplate the statement that Anti-D should only be used in pregnancy if the benefit outweighs the risk to the fetus. It is hard to evaluate the benefits and risks to a fetus when the fetus who is exposed to the possible risks of Anti-D will not experience any possible physical benefit from it. This is, in my experience, one of the main reasons why some of the women who decide to have Anti-D after birth or in response to a PSE in pregnancy have more questions and concerns when it comes to the decision about having routine antenatal Anti-D. I only wish we had better answers. At the time of writing, there have been no further studies and there continues to be a lack of interest in researching the long-term effects of antenatal Anti-D on unborn babies.

The dosage debate

The final issue I want to write about in this chapter relates to the data about how much Anti-D we should be offering and when. We know some things about that but, because the initial doses of 500iu (or 100µg of Anti-D and, in case you don't know, µg is the symbol for micrograms) that were chosen for the studies worked fairly well, those became the standard. These dosages were picked in a fairly arbitrary way, because in pioneering research one has to make educated guesses, and that's fair enough. But that does have consequences, because it is deemed unethical to give someone less than the standard once that standard has been set, so there has been very little research since then which could help refine our knowledge.

The history of how this happened further illustrates the way in which decisions relating to medicines tend to be made. In 1971, the authors of the World Health Organization Technical Report number 468 acknowledged that, *"There was little definite evidence, however, of general agreement on the value of any particular methods for defining the activity of preparations of this immunoglobulin and for prescribing dosage."* (WHO 1971: 16). The results of the initial dose trial that had been set up to consider this question were not published, as the researchers considered that they *"…added nothing material to those obtained in the main trial."* (Mollison *et al* 1974).

A larger trial then considered four different doses of Anti-D; 20µg, 50µg, 100µg and 200µg. About 200 women were in each of the dosage groups, and this trial was randomised and double blinded. The researchers acknowledge that the doses weren't exact. There were a few points where error could have occurred. They estimated that the amount of Anti-D in the phials was around 20 per cent higher than the dose stated in the study. The authors justified this by pointing out that it's not possible to inject the entire contents of the phial. In any case, the results failed to prove any differences between the effectiveness of the different doses, although the authors suggested that the dose of 20μg should be considered sub-optimal. So, in the absence of conclusive results, the standard dose of 500iu (or 100μg) was continued, and this remains the standard postnatal dose specified in the UK guidelines today. As I've mentioned, dosage varies around the world.

Howard *et al* (1997a) further considered the issue of dosage in relation to the European Committee for Proprietary Medicinal Products' (1992) suggestion that the routine administration of a larger postnatal dose of 1000-1500iu might eradicate the need for routine Kleihauer testing to determine whether a woman needed more than the standard dose of 500iu. While this suggestion might have been tabled as a cost-cutting exercise, a simple raising of the standard dosage of Anti-D may not offer satisfactory protection for all women. Howard *et al* (1997a) noted that this amount of Anti-D only cover a fetomaternal bleed of up to 15ml, and referred to the study by Mollison *et al* (1974) which showed that 0.3% of women experience a bleed greater than this amount. The fact that these women would be unprotected, while a much higher proportion of women would be exposed to far more Anti-D than they required, seems to suggest that this change is not beneficial. Despite this, some Hospital Trusts and Health Boards in the UK changed their guidelines to offer 1200iu as the standard postnatal dose. There are also a number who now give 1500iu as standard. When asked, several clinicians have told me that this is the only dose that they can access, although they are aware that other nearby units offer 500iu.

Reviewers have long noted that we don't have enough sound evidence concerning the optimal dose of Anti-D (Crowther & Middleton 1997, McBain *et al* 2015). While the doses given in Ireland, France and Canada are similar to those given in the UK, the standard dose in the USA is 1500iu (300μg). Several other European countries give 1000-1500iu, or 200-300µg (Howard *et al* 1997b). This is a large difference, with women in the USA and parts of Europe receiving three times the dose that women in other parts of the world receive. This also has implications in terms of cost, supply and the potential risk of side effects. It again reinforces that there was (and still is) much that we do not know.

While research in this area has dwindled of late, optimum Anti-D dosage remains an important consideration. Few people want to receive a higher dose of a medicine than they need, especially if this might increase the risk of experiencing side effects. This is also an important factor in the antenatal Anti-D debate. Why are we not seeing research exploring this question? Perhaps more importantly, why are we always so keen to find a dose that is optimal for the 'population,' rather than finding a way to work out the specific volume of Anti-D required by an individual? But the issue of availability, which I mentioned earlier in the book, comes into play again here. In many areas of the UK, midwives and doctors report that they are giving a standard dose of 1500iu because 500iu vials (which is the minimum recommended dose) of Anti-D are not available. The 1500iu doses are more expensive and they expose women and babies to a higher volume of a medicine made from blood than is deemed sufficient.

Where do we go from here?

I have, in this chapter, attempted to offer a thorough explanation of the research on which current guidelines are based. It is notable that there are gaps in this evidence. Much of the research is either of low quality or missing altogether. This is unfortunate, and it shows that the concerns of women and families have not been addressed. In the next chapter, I will widen the conversation in the hope of offering some thoughts for those who want to make decisions in spite of the state of the evidence.

4. The wider issues

The core problem that we face as far as our knowledge about Anti-D is concerned results from the beliefs and values which underpin health and maternity services. Those values in turn reflect the values of western culture more widely (Davis-Floyd 1992). The central concern relates to the question of who gets to make decisions about health and what kind(s) of knowledge and information are deemed important in that decision making. This is a key issue of our time. The increasing volume of information that is available to us is not helping. As I have also noted, the evidence we have focuses on short-term outcomes. It is based on a population-level approach. Groups consisting mostly of white, male, middle class, well-educated and well-meaning but often also paternalistic doctors, scientists and bioproducts company owners decided that all rhesus negative women with a rhesus positive baby should receive postnatal Anti-D.

The focus in that era was on preventing rhesus disease, and this was achieved. It was award winning, brilliant work. However, the results of the research also clearly showed that not all women need Anti-D because not all women would be sensitised without it. But there was no attempt to determine whether we could find out more and whether we could learn who could become sensitised, when and why.

This has happened in many other areas of health and maternity care as well. It results from the belief that it is okay for small groups of people to hold the power to make decisions regarding what larger groups of people should do, and what medicines or interventions they should be given. But it has subtle and frustrating effects on the knowledge that is available to those who want to consider all their options, or who would rather not have a routine intervention.

It's possible that we might not have been able to find out more about why most of the women who didn't have Anti-D didn't become sensitised. Even if we did know more, we would probably still only be able to offer probabilities and not certainties or guarantees. But then life doesn't tend to come with certainties or guarantees. The point is that no-one even tried to find out. When I came along and did just that, twenty years ago, my questions were met in some quarters with resistance, hostility and attempts to placate and silence me. (Clearly, that didn't work). To be fair, though, my questions were also welcomed by many, including some of those working at the heart of the establishment, who supported my work and used it as a means of proposing change.

Despite twenty years of awareness that questions and concerns exist, little has been done to address them. At the same time, the ethical framework which is a part of western medical culture effectively now ensures that some of these questions cannot be investigated. Even if we could find enough women to volunteer to be in trials (and I am confident, from the correspondence that I have received over the years, that this would be possible), any attempt to re-do some of those research studies and find out whether some groups of women are more or less prone to sensitisation would likely be blocked. The ethics committees who decide whether studies go ahead are sometimes dominated by those who have perpetuated the current problem, or who have a vested interest in the status quo. A member of a maternity services ethics committee shared her experience with me for this book, though she wished to remain anonymous:

"The ethics committee on which I sit is predominantly comprised of white, middle class, older men. Mostly doctors. They are dismissive of qualitative research and women's knowledge. Other voices may be present, but they are often in the minority and not listened to. Often, lay members don't have the knowledge to do more than ask basic questions about the ethics of a trial, and no attempt is

made to help them to learn or understand more, so there's little chance of being able to change anything. It's very frustrating."

Then there is the question of funding. This is problematic because our systems are set up to support research promoting intervention, drugs and technologies. It is almost impossible to gain funding for projects which challenge the status quo, or for which there is no financial benefit for the pharmaceutical or medical technology industries. This is why there is so much research into technologies and medicines and so little into the low-tech and freely available (or cheaply available or unpatentable) things that may make more of a difference.

Neither is there much chance of further research into the safety of Anti-D for women and/or unborn babies, although the concerns about potential risks of Anti-D and strength of feeling from some people would suggest that research is warranted. The environment of maternity care has undergone myriad changes since we began to offer postnatal Anti-D on a routine basis. While women giving birth in the early 1970s may not have felt they had much choice about their care, some of those giving birth in the twenty-first century are more active in demanding their rights. That is thanks in large part to the activist efforts of those who came before. The other significant change, of course, is that Anti-D is offered at other times as well now, and not just after a baby's birth.

In this chapter, I'm going to attempt to provide a bit more information and some alternative perspectives on a few different areas. Some of what I am discussing is speculative, theoretical and/or anecdotal, for all of the reasons I have just outlined. Until we can change the structures that underpin systems of maternity care, in some situations this is the best that we can offer. I'm going to look at issues relating to information, some alternative ideas and theories and then explore other aspects of the evidence in the hope of providing a wider perspective on some of the questions already raised.

Anti-D, women and families

Concerns have been expressed for years about how little involvement women and families have had in conversations about the Anti-D programme, and a handful of midwives and doctors have been very vocal about this. A British obstetrician raised questions about women's involvement in the rhesus programme in a letter to the British Medical Journal (Saha 1998). She conducted an *ad hoc* survey of 12 rhesus negative women who had received or been offered Anti-D. Not one knew that Anti-D was made from blood. They had assumed that it was either synthetic or from another natural source. Saha suggested it was imperative to inform women about the source of Anti-D and the chance of acquiring blood-borne infections. I later wrote about my own experience of this.

"When working as a hospital midwife, I noticed an interesting contrast between women who were offered blood transfusion and women who were offered Anti-D. Many women, when faced with the idea of receiving human blood, perhaps for lowered haemoglobin, will want to discuss whether they really need this, perhaps because they have concerns about viral transmission. By contrast, most women who are told they might benefit from Anti-D will simply accept this without questioning. Given that both products derive from human blood and carry similar risks, I can only assume that either women are keener to protect the health of their future babies than their own (which is entirely possible) or that they do not understand that Anti-D is a blood product." (Wickham 2005: 226).

Following the publication of Saha's letter, I conducted an *ad hoc* survey of eight obstetricians, and the results of that illustrate the other side of that problem (Wickham 2001). Not one of these doctors considered that women needed to know that Anti-D was made from blood. All but one felt women should 'not be made to worry' about such issues; Anti-D was (they argued) vital for the sake of a woman's future babies, and therefore women should 'do what doctors recommend' and 'not worry themselves' about the risk of infection. Over the years, I have been told by some obstetricians and obstetric organisations that lay women and consumer organisations would not understand the issues. Anti-D is a complex subject, they say, and the research is hard to understand. My response to this is usually to say that, of the more than 100 'lay' women who I have interviewed about Anti-D, and of the thousands of women, lay people and non-professional birth workers who I have taught over the years, not one has failed to understand the issues when they are explained well. Maybe the real reason women were excluded from decision making is that the paternalistic approach fails to perceive women as the focus of maternity care; treating them instead as vessels. Many obstetricians, like Saha, do not feel this way, of course. But prevailing patriarchal attitudes still underpin a lot of what happens today.

I have learned over the years that, while many midwives weren't given good information on Anti-D in their own pre-registration education, those who have later learned about the issues are usually keen to discuss Anti-D as an option rather than a given. And knowledge has improved with time. Twenty years ago, those working in systems of maternity care were less likely to possess the knowledge to support discussion with women and families than those working outside the system. When I first began to travel around the world and speak on this and other topics, I used to begin by asking midwives and birth educators what Anti-D was made from. Most were unaware it was made from blood. Some had never considered the question.

Today, knowledge and awareness has improved, but those working in systems of care instead report that, while they have the will and the desire to share full information with women and families, they are sometimes reprimanded (in direct and indirect ways) if they are seen to be offering the option to decline recommended interventions. Harkness *et al*

(2016: 500) also found that midwives, "...*were limited in their ability to fully engage with women in a process of individual informed decision-making, due partly to their own knowledge and understanding and partly to organisational culture and support.*" It's clear that we still have a long way to go.

What do women want?

Fyfe *et al* (2020) interviewed sixteen rhesus negative women in northern British Columbia and asked them about their experiences of the Anti-D programme.

"[We] *identified that RhD negative women are uninformed and want to be involved in the decision-making process regarding the prevention of RhD alloimmunization ... The participants in this study described lacking information regarding the prevention of RhD alloimmunization. They sought information to overcome the gaps in knowledge and a desire to be involved in the decision-making process.*" (Fyfe *et al* 2020).

Some of the direct quotes from participants in this study illustrate the nature of the issues that they encounter:

"*Two participants ... expressed they did not have a choice in receiving RhIG. It is unclear what the participants understood about RhIG is and why it is important, but RhDW05 said that she would have opted out of receiving RhIG if she knew her baby would be unaffected. The participant expressed frustration with the prevention program, stating that it was functioning under a worst-care* (sic) *scenario and utilized the phrase "just for kicks" to emphasize that the prevention seems unnecessary, particularly if some of the risk factors could be ruled out (like knowing the paternal Rh factor).*

[A participant said] *Well, it's like I'm negative so we didn't really know for sure if my husband was positive or negative, right, it was like test him when I get pregnant. So, with that they just like well cause we don't know, we're not going to test him, we're just going to assume that your baby is going to be positive and we're going to give you the, I can't remember what it's called. Whatever that shot is, midway through your pregnancy just for kicks, really, is how I felt about it."* (Fyfe *et al* 2020: e513).

It is clear that there's a problem here, and it is multifaceted. I documented my experience of receiving letters from women during my earlier research on this topic (Wickham 2001) and since. To clarify: I didn't invite such correspondence. Some women wrote spontaneously when they heard about my work. Here's what I wrote at the time:

"Altogether, 19 women made contact during the initial part of this research. All of them were rhesus negative, and most were concerned with the effects of and necessity for Anti-D – often because they had experienced unpleasant side effects from a previous dose. Several told me their immune systems had been moderately or severely compromised after receiving this product, and some were considering not having any more children because of the 'risk' of needing Anti-D again. None of the women who contacted me felt that they had received adequate information from their caregivers – this was often their prime reason for seeking further information and several stated that they did not even realise that they had a 'choice' in this area until afterwards." (Wickham 2001: 114).

I have now read and heard hundreds of similar messages, comments, letters and emails. Most of these describe problems that women and families have had trying to get adequate information. Some express concern about the robustness of the information they have been given. This occurs in two key and almost opposing ways. Some women feel that they are being given fear-based, over-medicalised information which over-promotes Anti-D and intervention and doesn't acknowledge their right to decide. A few, however, report not being able to get adequate detail from birth workers, and in some cases there is a tendency to underplay the possibility of sensitisation. My hope is that this book will help address both of those issues. But the reality is that the changes in attitude and improvements in education will only go so far. There remains the problem that we lack a lot of the information that women and families would benefit from having because that kind of knowledge and approach doesn't fit with modern, western cultural values, as I described at the beginning of this chapter.

Choice, control and coercion

Sadly, the issue of women not having enough choice and control in this area goes even deeper. I mentioned in chapter two that several thousand women in the German Democratic Republic (GDR) were infected with hepatitis C in a batch of contaminated Anti-D. This was not the only insult faced by this group of women:

"In the GDR, these women were compulsorily treated by physicians without sufficient information about the disease, diagnostics, and therapy. If the women refused medical care, they were coerced into it by the physicians. Medical care and research were inseparable. Without the knowledge of the women and without their consent, research was carried out on the blood samples and liver biopsies acquired from them. After the German reunification, the same physicians continued to conduct research on the same group of patients. Beginning in 1990, interferon therapy was offered to the women. Parallel to the medication with interferon, studies on the effects of the therapy were carried out. In this case as well, the women were not informed about the use of collected data, nor did they agree to it." (Schochow & Steger 2020: 127).

There are many areas of western medicine in which people – most notably women and Black and Brown people – have been abused, ignored and/or harmed. Some are very subtle, and the leaflets that are given out in many countries are an example of this. Some of the leaflets are produced by the companies that manufacture Anti-D. Others are published by medical organisations that take a paternalistic, technocratic, pro-intervention approach and do not involve women and families in the production of this information. Many leaflets justify why Anti-D is needed rather than presenting it as an option. Issues of choice are not mentioned and Anti-D leaflets and information websites are often decorated with pictures of smiling (and usually white) babies and blood cells. In fact, many of the leaflets only contain photos of white women and babies and give the statistics only for people of European descent without mentioning that the likelihood of a person being rhesus negative varies according to their ethnicity. (More on this in chapters one and five). While it is true that women of European descent are the most likely to be affected, it would perhaps be reassuring for women of Asian descent, for instance, to know that their chance of being rhesus negative is far lower than the leaflets suggest.

Most of the leaflets do not mention side effects. Many do not discuss the actual evidence. Even if they do, the reviews I have discussed in this book, which highlight the lack of robustness and certainty in some of the research, are not mentioned. Instead, some of the leaflets cite research carried out by the company producing the Anti-D. Such research is not usually publicly available, so it cannot be checked. It is thus impossible for women, families, midwives, doctors or other birth workers to evaluate the information given.

This is in stark contrast to the ideal. One midwife noted this in a letter written to a midwifery journal in response to a rather patronising article about Anti-D. The article did not acknowledge women's agency and repeatedly stated that Anti-D should be 'given' and not 'offered':

"Informed decision-making in relation to anti-D Ig is recognised as vital in relevant policy documents… The reasons for this are not

only that there are risks associated with anti-D Ig, both risk of blood-borne infection and of allergic reaction, but also that the benefits to women are impacted hugely by individual circumstances. For example, anti-D Ig is of absolutely no benefit to a woman who knows that her baby, or the father of her baby, is RhD negative. Similarly a woman who feels certain that this will be her final pregnancy may very reasonably choose to decline anti-D Ig." (Harkness 2015: 22).

It is my hope that some of the information in this chapter might add to the sparse information available. First, I want to return to address the question of responsibility.

The question of responsibility

I have previously discussed responsibility and noted that this is a contentious topic. On the one hand, if someone knows that they want to have Anti-D in one or more situations, taking personal responsibility in this area may mean that they are more likely to get it at the right time. On the other, there is an equally good argument that people should not have to take responsibility for such elements of their health care.

One report suggested that putting the responsibility on the woman can lead to Anti-D being missed. Cases of missed administration resulted from, *"Putting the onus on the woman to return for anti-D Ig when she is variously frightened, traumatised, too ill, or has her hands full with a new baby, instead of issuing it at presentation."* (Bolton-Maggs *et al* 2015: 97). This is an important point. However, there is a significant difference between putting the onus on someone who hasn't asked for it and who may not be in a position to take on anything else, and a situation where someone voluntarily opts to take responsibility for their own health. It's worth adding that we don't know (because no-one has ever measured this) how many doses of Anti-D have been given that might have been missed if a woman/family had not taken responsibility for this. There are many downsides to our modern approach of focusing on error and things going wrong. One of the biggest, is that we miss the opportunity to find out more about how things can go right.

In an ideal world, health care systems would be designed for maximum effectiveness in offering the right medicines and treatments to the right people at the right time. But we don't live in the ideal world, and this ideal relies on the very notion of standardisation that is at odds with the kind of care that women want from midwives and that midwives want to give (Kirkham 2018). It may be that we cannot have more agency without accepting more responsibility.

A holistic midwifery perspective on Anti-D

I have also carried out primary research on Anti-D (Wickham 2001). This was qualitative research, which involved talking to a small number of people to get in depth information about a topic. My study explored the knowledge and beliefs of 17 midwives from eight countries about the routine postnatal administration of Anti-D. Most of the midwives who participated in this study said they felt Anti-D was probably not necessary on a routine basis. Bear in mind that they were self-selected, though, so they already had views on this topic. But they also acknowledged that we don't currently have enough knowledge to be able to help all women work out whether they would become sensitised if they declined postnatal Anti-D.

Several of the midwives who participated in my research believed that there was much more to be known about the process of sensitisation, and they found it hard to believe that all rhesus negative women's bodies were failing in some way.

"I KNOW [participant's emphasis] *in my heart that anti-D is*

not necessary for all of these women. All of my experience as a midwife confirms to me that birth works. I just wish I knew why ... [and] exactly what affects this."

"I just find it incredibly hard to accept that there is such a huge loophole in such a sophisticated system."

"...if Anti-D is needed by some women, there must be a reason why. And if we can figure out the reason – on an individual basis – we might be able to learn more." (Wickham 2001: 64).

This shows the contrast between the midwifery and the obstetric viewpoint. The obstetric view focuses on the idea that all women's bodies might fail at any moment. Those who hold this view tend to seek universal things that can be done to everyone in the hope of controlling and reducing risk. A lot of trust is placed in technology and much less in women's bodies. The midwifery view is that women's bodies tend on the whole to work well, with occasional exceptions. Those who hold this view tend to express a need to simultaneously trust in physiology *and* to be vigilant for those exceptions. There's a further important point in the midwifery model, which is the idea that, when things do go awry, there tends to be a reason for that. If we can find the reason, we can sometimes predict issues and perhaps offer prevention measures or intervention to only that group of women. The prevention measures might be the same as those offered by proponents of western medicine, but they might also include things like nutrition, psychological interventions or, sometimes, holistic therapies. It's not that one of these views is inherently right or wrong; they are just different approaches. In reality, they both have merit and they are both, on occasion, problematic.

One of the key findings of the Wickham (2001) study was to do with the midwives' speculation about factors that they thought might increase the chance of sensitisation. These included some of the interventions that are commonly used in pregnancy and birth. That's not a new finding, and it is discussed elsewhere in the Anti-D literature. We have known for many years that medical intervention can cause harm, in a number of ways. We use the term iatrogenesis to describe harm caused by medical treatment. We talk about over-treatment or doing 'too much too soon' (Miller *et al* 2016) and 'cascades of intervention,' where one intervention leads to the need for another (Inch 1982). Davis-Floyd (1992) writes about the one-two punch, where technology that was developed to solve one problem leads to the need for further technology to solve problems caused by the first technology. Midwives in my study questioned whether even fewer women in the original clinical trials of Anti-D would have been sensitised if they had not been exposed to intervention that (the midwives speculated) may have caused their baby's blood to mix with their own. The irony here is that, at the time of writing this later version of my book, women who give birth in hospital in high-income countries often experience more intervention than the women who were in the Anti-D trials in 1969.

Some of the interventions named by the midwives as being possible causes of fetomaternal transfusion included ultrasound scans, exogenous oxytocin (i.e. the Syntocinon® or Pitocin® used in induction or augmentation of labour), artificial rupture of the membranes, amniocentesis and other invasive procedures involving the uterus. Some of these interventions have long been acknowledged as potentially sensitising events in the guidelines relating to Anti-D (Qureshi *et al* 2014). We have also long known that external cephalic version (Vos 1967, Stine *et al* 1985), caesarean section (du Bois *et al* 1991) and amniocentesis (Blajchman *et al* 1974, Lachman *et al* 1977) increase the likelihood of a fetomaternal transfusion.

The midwives in my study also speculated about whether some other interventions constitute potentially sensitising events. The interventions that they discussed included some that were an accepted part of medicalised maternity care, such as directed pushing and the use of local and epidural anaesthesia. The participants also discussed interventions that are known to be harmful but which are still used in some settings, such as fundal pressure. This is where a birth attendant pushes on the woman's abdomen in an attempt to speed the birth of the baby. The midwives' rationale for their concerns was that these interventions may threaten the integrity of the placenta and the structures which are designed to prevent the mother's and baby's blood from mixing. They suggested that directed pushing and fundal pressure might increase intrauterine pressure. The midwives also pointed out that epidural anaesthetic contains drugs that make blood vessels widen. They speculated that this might also increase the chance of sensitisation.

It would be useful to have studies to help confirm or refute these theories. But there are none. In addition, women who experience birth intervention rarely experience only one type of intervention, and few women currently decline interventions such as ultrasound scans. So it would be hard to do this research even in a cultural framework where the emphasis wasn't on population-level recommendations. A bigger problem is that, even if we can show that these interventions constitute PSEs, we can't know the effect of an absence of them on the chance of fetomaternal transfusion and/or sensitisation unless we do the studies that we already know we can't do. We do know for certain that the absence of intervention is no guarantee that sensitisation will not occur.

A number of things were discussed which the midwives thought might be worthy of research into whether they might offer some kind of protection, or perhaps enhance existing physiological mechanisms. Their ideas included ABO incompatibility (which I discuss below), nutrition, herbs and other substances thought to strengthen the placenta. They listed substances including bioflavonoids, magnesium, iodine, elderflower, red raspberry leaf and echinacea. Others wondered whether breastfeeding might play a role in protecting against sensitisation. It would be fascinating to know the method of feeding used by the women in the original trials and whether there was any correlation between the chance of sensitisation and feeding method. Could hormones released during breastfeeding play a part in suppressing antibody production? There is significant physiological communication between the mother's and baby's body during breastfeeding, so this would be a truly fascinating avenue for research. But the data on this were not made available in the original trials.

To my knowledge, citrus bioflavinoids are the only substances in the above list of suggestions that have been researched. Prior to the original Anti-D trials, researchers had suggested that these substances might strengthen placental attachment and increase the strength of blood vessels (Jacobs 1956, 1960, 1965). Jacobs' research also showed that these substances might improve the outcomes of babies born to women who had already become sensitised. The advent of Anti-D meant that this avenue was, like many others, ignored.

Going back to the science

While the midwives in the Wickham (2001) study offered a number of avenues which would be really interesting to explore, there is a need to remember that these are theories. They are based on experience, speculation, and belief. These ideas remain fascinating avenues down which we can only gaze in wishful hope that there was more interest in an approach that was more focused on women and families and less on population-based, technocratic ways of thinking.

It's important to understand the difference between a theory based on belief and experience and a theory which is also supported by evidence from well-designed research. Throughout this book, I have highlighted where the medical theories in this area are (and are not) supported by evidence, so in the next section I will do the same with the midwifery theories, and see if there is any evidence to support their viewpoint. But there is an important point to be made first.

As I have explained, quite a few elements of the current Anti-D programme are based on the experience, speculation and beliefs of obstetricians rather than on evidence from well-designed research studies. This kind of knowledge is called 'expert opinion' in some circles and colloquially termed 'GOBSAT' ('good old boys sitting around a table') in others. But it is essentially the same thing as the knowledge shared by the midwives in the Wickham (2001) study: theories developed by members of a particular occupational group who share a set of beliefs. But because our culture currently values medical knowledge as having more worth and authority than midwives' (or women's) knowledge, obstetricians' views are deemed to be expert opinion and are included in guidelines (Prusova *et al* 2014) while midwives' views generally are not. So many of these ideas have not been researched, although it is interesting that there is some evidence to support some of them, as I discuss below.

Back to transplacental bleeding

Midwives have long questioned whether transplacental bleeding is an inevitable part of birth, especially where birth is physiological and intervention has not taken place (Wickham 2001). They have also raised questions about the nature of the relationship between transplacental bleeding and sensitisation, which may be due to their belief that, on the whole, birth works well. So what does the evidence say?

It is clear from research that transplacental bleeding occurs more often than sensitisation, so we can be confident that the first does not automatically lead to the second. However, the rates of both of these occurrences vary widely between studies and our thinking has changed over time.

In Zipursky and Israels' (1967) study, fetal cells were seen in the blood of 17.6% of women. Two decades later, Bowman *et al* (1986) noted the passage of at least 0.01mL of fetal cells in 3%, 12%, and 46% of women in each successive trimester of pregnancy, though we don't know what sort of interventions the women were exposed to. Testing techniques and research methods have also improved significantly since these studies were done, but I haven't been able to find more recent, robust studies. Unfortunately, subsequent discussions of this issue in the haematology literature don't consider the question of whether or not pregnancy-related factors might influence the likelihood of this, as the midwives in my research suggested.

There is a bit of evidence to support their theory, though. One older study of the incidence of transplacental bleeding during curettage (a procedure in which a tool is used to remove anything in the womb) following abortion found that trauma to the uterus increased the chance of fetomaternal bleeding (Katz 1969). It is conceivable that a similar thing may occur from other procedures. Another small study (du Bois *et al* 1991) showed that fetomaternal haemorrhage was more likely to occur in instrumental delivery and caesarean section than in spontaneous birth. In that research, the rates of 'fetomaternal haemorrhage of clinical relevance' were 7.5% for spontaneous delivery, 11.1% for vacuum extraction and 17.7% for Caesarean section (du Bois *et al* 1991). We cannot know for sure, and it is very important not to mistake an association for a cause-and-effect relationship, but this does lend a bit of weight to the idea that more intervention may be associated with a higher chance of fetomaternal haemorrhage.

When it came to the rates of 'larger than average

fetomaternal bleed', however, these didn't differ between different types of birth. The number of women in du Bois *et al*'s (1991) study was relatively small (391), and we usually need larger numbers to see significant differences in things that occur less often, such as a larger than average fetomaternal bleed. It may also be inaccurate to consider the type of birth alone when other factors that could be associated with the type of birth such as the use of oxytocic drugs may (at least in theory) influence the chance of transplacental haemorrhage. We can see from the scientific literature in this area that there is an understanding that some medical procedures increase the chance of transplacental bleeding and thus sensitisation:

"Conditions increasing risks of alloimmunization correspond to increased fetal maternal hemorrhage, including miscarriage and termination of pregnancy, invasive diagnostic procedures, external version, Cesarean section, assisted vaginal delivery, surgical removal of the placenta, and transfusion for peripartum anemia." (Erickson 2020: 157).

None of this is concrete enough to inform advice that could be given to women and families who are wishing to limit the Anti-D they need, but it does suggest that there is more that could be learned about this topic.

Antibody formation

A few studies have looked at the percentage of rhesus negative people who form antibodies (in other words, become sensitised) to the D antigen after being transfused with rhesus positive red blood cells. Some studies have found that up to 80% of rhesus negative people will form anti-D antibodies if given significant volumes (200-500mls) of rhesus positive blood (Boctor *et al* 2003, Erickson 2020). However, there are reasons to be cautious about these figures and other studies have found lower rates of sensitisation (Erickson 2020). The high volumes of blood given in the studies that were set up to find out about sensitisation rates are far higher than the 4ml that is estimated to be the average amount of blood that might be involved in a fetomaternal bleed. But let's not forget that it is possible for a rhesus negative person to become sensitised after being in contact with a very small amount of rhesus positive blood (Erickson 2020). As I noted in chapter two, it is possible to become sensitised by sharing needles, so volume is not related to the chance of sensitisation in a simple fashion.

There are other reasons to be cautious about the idea that sensitisation rates are this high, and it may be helpful if I remind you at this stage that the likelihood of sensitisation among the rhesus negative women who took part in the original Anti-D trials was between 7.2% and 15% (see chapter three for more on this) and the rate of sensitisation before Anti-D was available in the USA is reported as being 14% (Moise 2002). In some of the studies I mentioned in the previous paragraph, participants were given more than one blood transfusion as the researchers were trying to induce sensitisation. And a number of other studies show lower figures, even with large volumes of blood transfused. For instance, Frohn *et al* (2003: 893) found that, *"...anti-D was detected in 16 of 78 patients..."* which is 20%. And Yazer & Triulz (2007) found a sensitisation rate of 13%, which is similar to the higher end of the range of results in the clinical trials of Anti-D. I have not found research suggesting a lower rate of sensitisation than this. Bear in mind that the studies do tend to be of those who had medically managed births, so we again have no way of knowing if less intervention would make a difference.

I will also note a few other important things. First, the immune system changes which occur during pregnancy may mean that data gathered from non-pregnant populations are meaningless. And the range of figures in these studies is so wide that these data are really not helpful at all. I have shared the detail not to annoy you with continued reminders of the uncertainty and lack of good research into this area, but to illustrate the variation in research findings and the uncertainties that are still under investigation. These include for instance, the question of why some people are more prone to become sensitised than others. Erickson (2020: 157) notes that, *"…transfusion recipients have been categorized as "non-responders," "responders," and "hyperresponders" based on their proclivity to alloimmunization."* She also notes that babies and children are less likely to become sensitised than adults; that sick and hospitalised people are more likely to become sensitised than healthy people; and people with thalassemia, sickle cell disease, and myelodysplastic syndromes are especially prone to becoming sensitised (Erickson 2020). If we can learn more about why these variations exist, we may be closer to helping those who want to make individualised decisions about Anti-D. But it is important to note that we still don't even know exactly why and how giving manufactured Anti-D works to prevent sensitisation from occurring.

I should also mention that, while the data in the original studies are incomplete, there is reason to think that the vast majority of research participants were white and of European descent. While it is true that this is the population who have the highest chance of being rhesus negative, the focus on this population means that we have little knowledge about whether people of different ancestry may be affected differently. Given that the rhesus factor is genetically determined, and that we know that some haemoglobino-pathies (or blood disorders that affect red blood cells) and certain other blood-related conditions are also genetically determined and thus more or less prevalent depending on ones' ancestry, this could be an important question.

ABO incompatibility

We do know a bit more about ABO incompatibility, which occurs where a woman has blood type O and her baby has blood type A or B. Although this can cause a mild form of HDFN, it's usually not serious (Erickson 2020). But, as recent research has confirmed, ABO incompatibility can confer some protection against sensitisation (Zwiers *et al* 2018, Erickson 2020). In simple terms, in situations where there is ABO incompatibility between mother and baby, the mother's antigens to A and B cells destroy any fetal blood that enters her circulation before it is possible for the body to recognise the D protein on the blood cells.

"The reduced rates of isoimmunization in Rh-negative mothers with ABO incompatibility were noted years ago in 1943 by Levine. More recent studies have demonstrated that the same protective effect of incompatibility extends to non-RhD isoimmunization, with lower rates than expected based on population at risk. This may be due to rapid clearance of the incompatible fetal cells from maternal circulation before an immunogenic response can be launched." (Erickson 2020: 151).

So we know that ABO incompatibility does confer some protection, but we have no way of quantifying this. And even if we could, there isn't much we can do with this knowledge unless we happen to also know the blood group of the unborn baby. As I have discussed elsewhere in the book, innovations in pregnancy testing offer a way forward when it comes to knowing whether a baby has the rhesus factor. But ABO incompatibility is another of those avenues that could continue to be explored and which might lead to us learning other useful things about blood groups, the rhesus factor, sensitisation and Anti-D.

The urge for change

There are calls from within the fields of birth and medicine for change, and for a more individualised approach to the Anti-D programme. It's always heartening to know that one is not alone in questioning things, so I have been particularly pleased to see the emergence of other voices joining those of us who have long tried to draw attention to this area. I welcome the studies that have looked more at women's and midwives' views and experiences, and I hope that we will see more of them. It has also been good to see the occasional voice in the medical literature, and also at medical conferences, who question the status quo.

There are areas which looked interesting, but which haven't been explored. One researcher documented the lamentable situation where at one point we had a possible alternative, and a safer form of Anti-D, but, *"...approaches faltered owing to the high costs of the large clinical trials necessary to show equivalent efficacy to an already highly effective approach."* (Franklin 2009: 1082). He concluded by arguing that, *"Serious thought must be given now to whether we should still be giving human-derived plasma products to healthy people in 10, 20, or 50 years time, when viable alternatives remain unexplored."* (Franklin 2009: 1082).

On the other hand, innovations in fetal rhesus testing mean that we can now identify the 42% of rhesus negative women who are carrying a rhesus negative baby and thus do not need to think about whether they wish to have Anti-D during or after their current pregnancy. This is partly thanks to a number of researchers and reviewers from around the globe. They have argued that targeted antenatal Anti-D, by which we mean offering this only to women whose babies are rhesus positive, is an effective, cost-effective and woman-centred approach to giving antenatal Anti-D (Teitelbaum *et al* 2015, Neovius 2016, de Haas 2016, Darlington *et al* 2018,

Runkel *et al* 2020). We also know that a targeted approach to offering Anti-D is effective where a woman has had an induced abortion (Jensen *et al* 2019). This is the most woman-centred innovation in the Anti-D programme in recent years. That's because the testing, which is now being rolled out in many countries, will save hundreds of thousands of doses being given unnecessarily each year. In the UK, I estimate that offering fetal rhesus testing to all pregnant women, either as a stand-alone test or as part of the NIPT test that I discussed in chapter two, will save 40,000 women a year from having unnecessary Anti-D.

As I write, fetal rhesus testing programmes are still being rolled out. But many countries have plans to bring testing programmes online and to ultimately offer this to all rhesus negative women. For the 42% of rhesus negative women who are carrying a rhesus negative baby, this will be game-changing. It is important not to forget that the 58% of rhesus negative women who are carrying a rhesus positive baby will still need to carefully weigh up their options when it comes to whether or not they wish to have Anti-D. There is also, as I have already noted, a need to ensure that all the possible downsides of testing are discussed so that individuals can make an informed decision. This is especially the case where fetal rhesus testing is only offered as part of a wider NIPT programme, where other things will be tested for as well.

Ultimately, the decision is down to the individual, and so I want to return, in the last part of this chapter, to a wider question. Throughout this book, I have analysed the research and thinking that has been carried out on the topic of Anti-D. What can all of this analysis offer to those who want to make individualised decisions about Anti-D?

What's right for you?

As I noted at the beginning of this book, all interventions have pros and cons, and it's a question of being able to weigh them up within the light of your individual context. It's also the case that you might want an intervention, drug or product in one situation, but perhaps not in another. Some women for instance, are happy to have postnatal Anti-D and to consider it, depending on the circumstances, if they have a PSE during pregnancy, but they do not want to have Anti-D given routinely in pregnancy. Some women want Anti-D at every opportunity. Others decide to have it after one or two births but, when they reach a point where they know that the current pregnancy is their last and they don't plan on any more babies, then they decline it. Thanks to the advent of fetal rhesus testing, some now know whether their baby is rhesus positive or negative before they have to consider Anti-D. In some countries where fetal rhesus testing is not yet freely available, I know couples who have paid for antenatal testing of their baby's blood group in the hope that they are one of those who will get some certainty from knowing that their baby is rhesus negative. There are other families who get the baby's father-to-be tested before they even become pregnant. These are merely examples though, and I haven't even covered the full range of options.

You now know the key things about Anti-D and why it is offered. So I will summarise some of the key points, and then offer a few pointers to key issues that women and families may wish to consider when thinking about this area.

- Fetomaternal bleeding and sensitisation aren't inevitable, but a rhesus negative woman who gives birth to a rhesus positive baby has about a one in eight chance of becoming sensitised if she does not have postnatal Anti-D: more in chapters one and three.

- Becoming sensitised means that there is a chance that, if a woman later becomes pregnant with a rhesus positive baby, the baby may become ill during pregnancy and need treatment, both during pregnancy and after birth. If future babies are rhesus negative, they will not be affected. More in chapter one.

- Most affected babies will have a mild or moderate form of rhesus disease. All affected women will be offered screening, and some babies will be deemed to need treatment, either during pregnancy and/or after birth. A few babies who have HDFN (and we unfortunately do not know the exact proportion) will be severely affected. In high-income countries, around 96 per cent of babies who are severely affected by HDFN now survive, but up to one in 25 will sadly die. Key terms are explained in chapter one, and the research relating to this is discussed in chapters three and four.

- It is also possible to become sensitised at other points during pregnancy, and Anti-D is also offered (and in some areas recommended) in several other situations. We do not have enough evidence to say with any certainty what the likelihood of sensitisation is in different situations, whether Anti-D is effective in these situations and how many women need to be given Anti-D in order to save one baby's life. In the case of routine antenatal Anti-D, we need to give routine Anti-D to thousands of women to prevent one death from HDFN: see chapters three and four for more on this.

- Anti-D is a medicine made from blood. It has possible side effects and downsides which need to be weighed up against the benefits that it offers: see chapters two and three for much more detail on the downsides and side effects of Anti-D.

- Because Anti-D is all about protecting future babies, a woman who knows for sure that her current baby (or next baby, if this is something that you are considering ahead of time) will be her last baby may wish to take that into account in making her decision. That includes anyone who is having a hysterectomy or permanent contraception as part of their birth. In this situation, contraception is a key consideration.

- Women who wish to have Anti-D in one or more situations may also wish to take responsibility for knowing the situations when this is recommended in their area of the world and, if necessary, be prepared to ask about it, or ask for it. Bear in mind, that no matter how well intentioned individual health professionals are, the fragmentation that is a part of many systems of maternity care may mean that this gets overlooked. So do not be afraid to ask about Anti-D any time you have any concern, or think you should be offered this: see chapters one and two for details and examples.

- Women who do not wish to have Anti-D (or who do not wish to have more Anti-D than they really need) can do a number of things to gain more information before having to make decisions. If you know you are rhesus negative, you may wish to find out whether the baby's father is rhesus positive or negative. More on how to do this in chapter five, but the quickest, cheapest and nicest way to do this is if he donates blood. If you're lucky and he is rhesus negative you won't have to think about any of this. The chances of the baby's father being rhesus negative will vary depending on his ancestry: more on this in chapter five as well.

- Even if a baby's father is rhesus positive, there is still a chance that the baby will be rhesus negative. This depends on genetics: see chapter five. If that's the case then you might want to ask locally about the options for finding this out, and consider whether that is something you would want to do. More on this in chapter two.

- In many areas, fetal rhesus testing is now available, although this may need to be paid for privately. It will become an option in more areas over the coming years. This enables parents to know whether their baby is rhesus positive or rhesus negative. If the baby is rhesus negative, then Anti-D does not need to be given at any point during pregnancy or after birth: more on this in chapter two.

- Although this is not a common option, I will mention that I have met one or two women who felt so strongly that they did not wish to have Anti-D that they declined it on the basis that they would get their antibodies tested six months after their baby's birth and then, if they had become sensitised, would choose to not have future babies. In this situation, such testing is likely to need to be paid for privately, even in countries where health care is free at the point of access.

- Parents who are seeking assisted fertility treatment and who have concerns about this area may wish to talk to their care provider about issues relating to Anti-D before they have treatment. Innovations such as pre-implantation diagnosis may be offered to women who have been sensitised. As with all interventions and tests, the pros and cons need to be carefully weighed up.

- As with many areas of birth-related decision making, different people have very different beliefs and values. What's really important is that you and your family are able to get good enough information to understand the issues. You can then use the information to make the decisions that are right for you.

5. Frequently asked questions

In this chapter, I briefly answer some of the key questions that I get asked about Anti-D and expand a bit on a few areas that were a bit too detailed to fit in to the flow of the chapters. There's a bit of repetition here, and I make no apology for that. It's so that people can find the information they need quickly if they are in a hurry.

How do rhesus groups relate to genetics?

I haven't discussed genetics and blood types at length in this book, but there are a few things that are worth knowing. The gene for making rhesus negative blood is recessive and the gene for making rhesus positive blood is dominant. This means that anyone who is rhesus negative themselves will always have two rhesus negative genes. Otherwise, the dominant rhesus positive gene would dominate and they would be rhesus positive. A rhesus negative person can only ever pass on a rhesus negative gene to their baby; they have two of those so that's the only kind they can pass on. So a rhesus negative mother and a rhesus negative father can only ever have rhesus negative babies. As long as the woman doesn't receive rhesus positive blood from another source, she won't have to make decisions relating to Anti-D because there will be no need to even offer it.

A rhesus positive person, however, might have two rhesus positive genes (we call this homozygous rhesus positive), or they might have one rhesus positive and one rhesus negative gene (heterozygous rhesus positive). There are blood tests which can tell if someone is homozygous or heterozygous rhesus positive, but (at the time of writing) this can't be determined from the sort of tests carried out in health care.

If a person is heterozygous rhesus positive and they pass on the rhesus negative gene to their rhesus negative partner, their baby will be rhesus negative. That's because two rhesus negative genes equals a rhesus negative baby. If the rhesus positive partner passes on the rhesus positive gene, the baby will be rhesus positive because this gene is the dominant one.

So it is genetically possible that a heterozygous rhesus positive father can create rhesus positive and rhesus negative babies with a rhesus negative woman. But a homozygous rhesus positive father can only father rhesus positive babies. This is useful to know in some ways, but it's a moot point in others, because it isn't possible for the vast majority of people to find out their exact genetic make-up. It's important to know though, that a rhesus negative mother who is pregnant by a rhesus positive partner may have a rhesus positive or a rhesus negative baby: with a heterozygous partner, the chance is 50:50 depending on which gene the father passes on.

How are rhesus groups affected by ancestry?

I could (though I probably won't) write another whole book about rhesus groups and ancestry, as many fascinating theories exist about this. Scientists and anthropologists have put forward several possible theories to explain why there are far more rhesus negative people in Europe and in people of European descent than in people whose ancestors come from some other parts of the world. We don't yet know which, if any, of these are true. Some non-scientists have rather wilder theories which you can, if you're interested, find online.

What we do know, is that someone's chance of being rhesus positive or negative is dependent on their ancestry. That's because it is genetically determined. Some of what we know about this comes from older research or just what scientists, midwives and doctors see in the results of laboratory tests. Modern studies tend to focus more on the actual genes rather than how they are expressed in blood groups.

We know, for instance, that the incidence of the rhesus negative blood type is far lower in Aboriginal people, Torres Strait Islanders, Maori and Pacifica people than in people of European descent who now live in Australia and New Zealand. We think that the chance of someone from one of the former groups being rhesus negative is about 1%. We also believe that the chance of being rhesus negative is about 1% for people of Asian descent, about 8% for people of African ancestry, about 15% for most people of European ancestry and up to 30-35% for people with ancestors from the Basque region (Bowman 1992).

It's important to remember that this only gives us a rough idea of how *likely* someone might be to have a particular rhesus factor. The only way of knowing whether you are rhesus positive or rhesus negative is through a blood test.

Do I need a Kleihauer test alongside Anti-D?

There is some variation in what is offered and when. In some countries, Kleihauer testing would not be offered in a situation where someone's medical history and/or the clinical signs clearly indicate that this would not be necessary. One example is a PSE in early pregnancy in a country that offers Anti-D before 12 weeks, but where it is clear that the dose of Anti-D given is more than adequate for the amount of blood that could have entered the maternal bloodstream. Kleihauer testing is also not offered alongside routine antenatal Anti-D.

Once a certain point in pregnancy has been reached (and this is generally considered to be 12 weeks, but it may vary a bit depending on where you are in the world), most women will be offered a Kleihauer test alongside a dose of Anti-D if they experience a PSE. You can always decline a Kleihauer test, or any other kind of test. But if you decide you want to have Anti-D after a PSE, it's a really good idea to have a Kleihauer test (or whatever is offered in your area) as well.

As I explained in chapter two, a Kleihauer test will determine whether more fetal blood cells have passed into the maternal circulation than can be cleared by a standard dose of Anti-D. Without a Kleihauer test, we can't be sure that we are giving an effective dose of Anti-D.

Having said that, I have lived and worked in rural and remote areas of the world where sometimes it's just not possible to do a Kleihauer within the necessary timeframe. In that case, Anti-D may be given without a Kleihauer test.

How many women will be offered more than the standard dose of Anti-D?

Estimates of this vary, partly because the standard dose is different in different areas. Moise (2002) suggests that about one in 1000 women are found to have a larger fetomaternal transfusion than will be cleared by a standard dose of Anti-D. Some hospital-based laboratory scientists have told me that their estimate would be closer to one in 100.

There are other possible reasons for this discrepancy. One is that different testing measures and standards are used in different areas. It may also be that more women have larger fetomaternal bleeds in areas where there is more medical intervention.

If Anti-D hasn't been given within 72 hours, is there any point in having/giving it?

The 72 hour window for giving Anti-D after a potentially sensitising event derived from some of the early research studies. As is often the case, researchers needed to pick a 'window' of time for their protocol, and they chose 72 hours. This has become the standard of care because Anti-D worked when given within that time window. Certainly it is best to give it sooner rather than later. But it is now acknowledged that, *"If, exceptionally, this deadline has not been met some protection may be offered if anti-D Ig is given up to 10 days after the sensitising event."* (Qureshi *et al* 2014). Some sources say that it is worth giving even if 13 or more days have passed, but it is less likely that it will be effective if antibody formation has begun.

Can I have Anti-D at the same time as a vaccine?

Anti-D shouldn't be given at the same time as a live vaccine. Anti-D should always be the higher priority because it is time sensitive. Generally, the recommendation is to wait three months after the administration of Anti-D before having a live vaccine. The issue is that the Anti-D may prevent the vaccine from working. It would be wonderful if all doctors, midwives and birth workers knew and considered this, but that has not been my experience. Often, vaccines are offered routinely and without thought for whether anything may interfere with them. If you are offered a vaccine that you wish to have and you have recently had Anti-D, or are likely to have Anti-D in the near future, you may wish to discuss this with your health care provider. If they do not know about this, I suggest that you show them this book and also ask them to look at the Anti-D product insert as well as the vaccine product information, as many contain information about this.

Check the vaccine to find out if it is live, inactivated or another type of vaccine. On the whole, vaccines for measles, mumps, rubella, chickenpox, smallpox, rotavirus and yellow fever are live. Flu, hepatitis A, whooping cough and polio vaccines tend to be inactivated. At the time of writing, no COVID-19 vaccine contains live virus. There are other types of vaccines too, so always check the product information or ask a midwife or doctor. If in doubt, and if there is no urgency, it may be better to wait to ensure maximum protection.

I was given Anti-D after a PSE in pregnancy; will I still be offered routine antenatal Anti-D?

In most areas, including the UK, yes. It's up to you whether or not you decide to have it, of course, but the rationale for offering it is that the Anti-D that you were given for the potentially sensitising event may have been used up.

The theory is that routine antenatal Anti-D is given to cover you and protect against possible 'silent' sensitisation through the last few weeks of pregnancy. More on routine antenatal Anti-D and silent sensitisation in chapter three.

How can we find out someone's rhesus factor?

There are a number of ways to do this. For instance if you want to know your own rhesus factor before becoming pregnant or if you want to work out the baby's father's rhesus factor. The person's GP surgery may be able to tell you, if they have it on file, or you may be able to find it out from medical notes and letters that have been sent in the past. Depending on someone's age, their own mother may know, or it may be written in a baby book or child health record. Many parents keep these for a long time!

If you can't find an existing record of it, there are other options. If you want to know about the baby's father's rhesus factor, it is worth asking your midwife or doctor whether having the baby's father's blood tested is an option in your area. It often isn't or, if it is, you may have to pay, but sometimes people get a positive response, especially if you explain that you are keen to avoid Anti-D if the baby's father is rhesus negative. One quick, easy, free and altruistic way of finding out someone's blood group and rhesus factor in many countries is to go and donate blood. You do have to fit the donation centre's criteria though, so check these before going.

The other option that some people can access is using an Eldon card. These are special cards that are made by a Danish company (www.eldoncard.com) and used by health care providers to find out someone's blood and/or rhesus factor quickly. They are for instance, used in blood banks, by the military, and in some emergency situations where the identity of the patient may not be clear. These are now, like almost anything, fairly easily available on the internet. But please ensure you undertake adequate research if you explore this option, and you ensure that you know exactly what you are buying and from whom. This is one time when you *really* don't want to buy a cheap imitation. And do read the instructions carefully before you begin.

My rhesus factor has changed! What's going on?

While not common, this isn't as rare as you might think. Over the years, I've heard from many women (and a few men) who were once told that they were rhesus negative, only to later find out that they are rhesus positive. Sometimes it happens the other way around.

There are a few reasons this might happen. The first is that an error occurred in the testing which meant that the results you were given on one of the occasions were incorrect. In the past, blood tests were less sensitive than they are now. You might have been told that you were rhesus positive but you're really rhesus negative, or you might have been told that you're rhesus negative when you're actually rhesus positive. It's frustrating but mistakes happen, and they may result from a fault with the technology or from human error.

But there is a second, more likely situation in which you might be told on different occasions that you have a different rhesus factor. I have so far only mentioned two rhesus types – positive and negative. While I did this for the sake of clarity in the book, there are also some other quite rare possibilities.

A very few people have a rhesus type called weak D. In the past, this type was also known as D^u and you might see that term if you come across old maternity or medical notes. We say that someone is 'weak D' when they are rhesus positive but they have fewer D antigens on their red blood cells than normal. This blood type is found in 0.2% to 1% of people of European descent, and is thought to be genetically determined (Wagner *et al* 1999). It is even rarer in people from other parts of the world. There's also another possibility, which is that someone can be 'partial D', which has also been called 'D mosaic' and 'D variant'.

The science that underpins this is beyond the scope of this book, but I have included a couple of explanations and references for those who are interested in learning more:

"Blood that is D- and D^u-positive with anti-D has been classified by Tippett; such blood types lack part of the D mosaic and are considered to be "D variants" yet are typed routinely as Rh positive." (White *et al* 1983: 1069).

As above, more sensitive blood tests exist these days, so a more recent test might highlight a variant which wasn't previously spotted. Erickson (2020) describes the current state of knowledge and practice in this area:

"Individuals identified as partial D should be treated as Rh-negative patients and Rh positive blood donors to prevent inadvertent exposure and alloimmunization. These mothers should receive anti-D-immune globulin, as their fetus may inherit the fragment of D antigen they lack. Individuals identified as weak D should be treated as Rh-positive patients and blood donors, as any amount of D antigen can induce immunization in Rh-negative blood recipients. The confirmed weak D mother does not need RhIg administration." (Erickson 2020: 151).

There have also been some very rare cases where somebody's blood type actually changed. These have been associated with very unusual situations, for instance having leukaemia (Chérif-Zahar *et al* 1998).

This is a complex situation. If this happens to you, and you need to make a decision about Anti-D or any other aspect of your care, talk to your midwife or other caregiver. If they are not knowledgeable about this specific issue (which they may well not be, as it's a specialist area) then you may wish to ask for a referral to a haematologist so you can chat through your individual circumstances and what this means for you.

Does Anti-D contain mercury or latex?

Not these days, no. In the past, there have been concerns that a mercury-based preservative called thimerosal was used in some preparations of Anti-D. At the time of publication, none of the preparations of Anti-D used in the western world contain thimerosal. None of the Anti-D delivery systems that I am aware of contain latex; a substance that some people have a severe allergic reaction to. Latex allergy is now well understood in most countries.

If you have any concerns about what is in Anti-D or any other drug or product that you are offered, you can ask to see the product information leaflet before you decide whether or not you want it. It is also very easy these days to do an internet search on drugs and products to see what they contain. Just ensure that you are looking at the product information or a site run by pharmaceutical professionals such as Drugs.com. There are, sadly, a number of people who spread harm through conspiracy theories about medicines such as Anti-D and vitamin K. And some of the information that can be found on the internet is worryingly untrue.

In conclusion

Like many preventative interventions, Anti-D can be life-saving. But nothing comes with a guarantee and no medicine or intervention is without downsides and cost. Like all birth-related decisions, the decision about whether and when to have Anti-D and the tests that relate to this need to be weighed up and considered in the light of one's individual situation. With Anti-D, this is not just one decision. Some women and families opt to have Anti-D in some situations and not others. There is no right or wrong path. There's only the path that's right for you and your family.

I began this book by sharing the story of my research into Anti-D and the fact that the publication of this book marked the fiftieth anniversary of the Anti-D programme and the twentieth anniversary of my original work on this topic. So it seems only fitting to take a step back and consider what has changed in the past twenty years.

On a positive note, some key areas of our thinking and understanding have been refined. The advent of fetal rhesus testing has meant that the 42% of rhesus negative women who are carrying a rhesus negative baby can now find this out, which means they will know early in pregnancy that they don't need to think further about Anti-D. It is also good to see reviewers acknowledging the poor quality of some of the research which underpins recommendations in this area.

Disappointingly little else has changed. Acknowledging the poor quality of the trials which are the basis for some elements of the Anti-D programme is a bit hollow given that there has been no related drive to undertake better research. Neither have there been moves to review guidelines that are not informed by the evidence and that have caused concern.

As in many areas of research, there has been a serious lack of attention to what women and families want, and what their priorities are. This is not because obstetricians and midwives aren't concerned about these things. Over the last twenty years I have had countless conversations with hundreds of people from both professions, and many of them share my (and perhaps now your) concerns about the lack of good knowledge that can help people making the decisions that are right for them. The problems are more structural. They exist in relation to the priorities of modern society, and to the way that research is funded and carried out. They reflect the wider values of our culture. And while those values very much prioritise the idea of individual choice in some ways, in other areas of life (with maternity care being a great example) we actually have an increasingly narrow range of choices, even if it appears otherwise. Many people find themselves being led down a path which is not necessarily the one they would have chosen for themselves.

While I was researching this book, a quote from one of the midwives in my original study really struck me:

"Do you remember that line in Jurassic Park, where the mathematician says to the scientists who've regenerated dinosaurs, 'You were so busy trying to find out if you could, that you didn't stop to think about whether you should.'" (Wickham 2001: 70).

With Anti-D and some other birth interventions, it's not so much that we ought have stopped to ask whether we 'should,' because it's very clear that Anti-D and the Anti-D programme has helped many people. It's more that a relatively small group of people saw one route to the desired destination and decided that we should all go that way and remain on the same path. Those people had a very particular set of beliefs about the world, about maternity care, about the female body and about the right of women to make their own decisions. You may or may not share their beliefs.

There were, and still are, other avenues which might get us to the same destination. Now that we have learned more, these avenues may even be better, or they might at least have fewer hazards along the way, but these other possible routes remain unmapped. And, to take the analogy further, there is a ban on map-making. Those who chose the path have deemed it unethical to research other options, because their path works. It's still possible to take the alternative routes, but we can't tell you how likely it is that they will take you where you want to go. Information on what you might find has been limited by the focus on everybody taking the one road.

While I wish that I was able to offer more certainty and better data, I hope that the contents of this book have helped you to understand the issues relating to Anti-D more clearly and provided a bit of a map. I hope I have helped make clear the parts of the issue where we do have some data and numbers that we can use as a basis for decision making. I also hope that, even though we are still left with uncertainties, the very act of naming and discussing the uncertainties can make it a bit easier to think about how we can navigate and live with them. I hope that this book will enable you to weigh up the different options and data (where available) in relation to your personal circumstances and to make the decisions that are right for you.

To keep in touch and see more of Sara's work:

Sign up for my free newsletter and get information on
my books, courses and other projects at
www.sarawickham.com/news

If you have enjoyed this book and found it useful,
please leave a review at your favourite book retailer –
it really helps highlight it to others who might need it.

Other books by Sara which you might enjoy:

Plus Size Pregnancy: what the evidence really says about
higher BMI and birth

In Your Own Time: how western medicine controls the start
of labour and why this needs to stop

Inducing Labour: making informed decisions

Group B Strep Explained

Vitamin K and the Newborn

What's Right For Me? Making decisions in pregnancy and
childbirth

Birthing Your Placenta: the third stage of labour

101 tips for planning, writing and surviving your
dissertation

References

ACOG (2017). Practice Bulletin No 181: Prevention of Rh D Alloimmunization. Obstetrics & Gynecology 130(2): e57-70.

Akers C, Glazebrook B, Bielby L *et al* (2019). RhD Immunoglobulin: Are we following the guidelines? Women and Birth 32(1): S30.

Akers C, Savoia H, Kane S *et al* (2018). Misinterpretation of blood group and antibody screen leading to serious errors in RhD immune-globulin administration. ANZJOG 59(1): 161-64.

Al-Kubaisy W, Daud S, Al-Kubaisy MW *et al* (2018). Maternal hepatitis C (HCV) infection and Anti-D immunoglobulin therapy: study testing antibodies, RNA and Genotype of HCV in Baghdad. The Journal of Maternal-Fetal & Neonatal Medicine 32(20): 3464-69.

American College of Obstetricians and Gynecologists (1999). Prevention of Rh D alloimmunization: clinical management guidelines for obstetricians and gynecologists. IJGO 66(1): 63-70.

Bennebrock Gravenhorst J (1989). Rhesus isoimmunisation. In: Chalmers I *et al* (Eds). Effective Care in Pregnancy and Childbirth. Oxford University Press: Oxford. 565-77.

Blajchman NI, Maudsley RF, Uchida I *et al* (1974). Diagnostic amniocentesis and fetomaternal bleeding. Lancet I: 993-94.

Boctor FN, Ali NM, Mohandas K *et al* (2003). Absence of D-alloimmunization in AIDS patients receiving D-mismatched RBCs. Transfusion 43: 173-76.

Bolton-Maggs PHB (Ed), Poles D *et al* (2015) on behalf of the Serious Hazards of Transfusion (SHOT) Steering Group. The 2014 Annual SHOT Report.

Bowman JM (1978). Preventing Rh sensitisation during pregnancy. Perinatal Care 2:24–32.

Bowman JM, Pollock JM, Penston LE (1986). Fetomaternal transplacental hemorrhage during pregnancy and after delivery. Vox Sang 51: 117-21.

Bowman JM (1992). Maternal alloimmunization and fetal hemolytic disease. In: Reece EA *et al* (eds). Medicine of the Fetus and Mother. Philadelphia: JB Lippincott.

Bowman JM (1998). RhD hemolytic disease of the newborn. NEJM 339: 1775-77.

Bowman JM and Pollock JM (1978). Rh isoimmunisation during pregnancy: antenatal prophylaxis. CMAJ 118: 623-27.

Chan N, Smet M-E, Sandow R *et al* (2017). Implications of failure to achieve a result from prenatal maternal serum cell-free DNA testing: a historical cohort study. BJOG 125(7): 848-55.

Chérif-Zahar B, Bony V, Steffensen R *et al* (1998). Shift from Rh-positive to Rh-negative phenotype caused by a somatic mutation within the RHD gene in a patient with chronic myelocytic leukaemia. Brit J Haematology 102(5): 1263-70.

Choate JD (2018). ABO and Rh Blood Groups. In: Maitta RW (2019). Clinical Principles of Transfusion Medicine. Elsevier. 15-24.

Clarke CA, Donahoe WTA & McConnell RB (1963). Further experimental studies on the prevention of Rh haemolytic disease. BMJ 1: 979-84.

Clutterbuck H (1838). Dr Clutterbuck's Lectures On Bloodletting: Lecture 1. The London Medical Gazette.

Coombes R. (1999). Midwives cautioned over risks of using untested blood product. Nursing Times, 95(24): 7.

Crowther C & Middleton P (1997). Anti-Rh-D prophylaxis postpartum. In: Pregnancy and Childbirth Module of the Cochrane Database of Systematic Reviews. Neilson JP *et al* (Eds). The Cochrane Collection, Issue 4, Oxford, Update Software 1997.

Darlington M, Carbonne B, Mailloux A *et al* (2018). Effectiveness and costs of non-invasive foetal RHD genotyping in rhesus-D negative mothers: a French multicentric two-arm study of 850 women. BMC Pregnancy and Childbirth 18: 496.

Davis-Floyd R (1992). Birth as an American Rite of Passage. University of California Press.

de Crespigny L & Davison G (1995). Anti-D administration in early pregnancy – time for a new protocol. ANZJOG 35: 385-87.

de Haas M, Thurik FF, van der Ploeg CPB *et al* (2016). Sensitivity of fetal *RHD* screening for safe guidance of targeted anti-D immunoglobulin prophylaxis: prospective cohort study of a nationwide programme in the Netherlands. BMJ 355:i5789.

Drugs.com (2020a). D-Gam Anti-D Side Effects. www.drugs.com/sfx/d-gam-anti-d-side-effects.html

Drugs.com (2020b). Rho (d) immune globulin pregnancy and breastfeeding warnings www.drugs.com/pregnancy/rho-d-immune-globulin.html

du Bois A, Quaas L, Lorbeer H *et al* (1991). Fetomaternal transfusion in relation to mode of delivery. (in German). Zentralblatt fur Gynakologie 113(17): 927-33.

Dumasia A, Kulkarni S & Joshi SH (1989). Women receiving anti-Rho(D) immunoglobulin containing HIV antibodies. Lancet II (8660): 459.

Durandy A, Fisher A & Griscelli C (1981). Dysfunctions of pokeweed mitogen-stimulated T and B lymphocyte responses induced by gamma globulin therapy. J Clinical Investigation 67: 867.

Edwards N & Wickham S (2018). Birthing your placenta: the third stage of labour. Avebury: Birthmoon Creations.

Erickson ML (2020). Alloimmunization in Pregnancy. In: Maitta RW (Ed). Immunologic Concepts in Transfusion Medicine. Elsevier. 149-165.

European Committee for Proprietary Medicinal Products (1992). Note for guidance: core summary of product characteristics for human anti-D immunoglobulin, im. Brussels: Commission of European Communities, 1992. (111(3463/92-EN.)

Finning K, Martin P, Summers J *et al* (2008). Effect of high throughput RHD typing of fetal DNA in maternal plasma on use of anti-RhD immunoglobulin in RhD negative pregnant women: prospective feasibility study. BMJ 336:816.

Franklin IM (2009). Prevention of rhesus haemolytic disease of the fetus and newborn. Lancet 373(9669): 1082.

Frohn C, Dumbgen L, Brand JM *et al* (2003). Probability of anti-D development in D- patients receiving D+ RBCs. Transfusion 43: 893-98.

Fyfe TM, Ritchey MJ, Taruc *et al* (2014). Appropriate provision of anti-D prophylaxis to RhD negative pregnant women: a scoping review. BMC Pregnancy and Childbirth 14: 411.

Fyfe TM, Lavoie JG, Payne GW *et al* (2020). Rhesus D factor (RhD) negative women's experiences with pregnancy: An interpretive description. Women and Birth 33(6): e511-e518.

Garvey P, Murphy N, Flanagan P *et al* (2017). Disease outcomes in a cohort of women in Ireland infected by hepatitis C-contaminated anti-D immunoglobulin during 1970s. J Hepatology 67(6): 1140-47.

Gaskin IM (1989). Rethinking Rhogam. Birth Gazette, 6(1).

Ghosh S & Murphy WG (1994). Implementation of the rhesus prevention programme: a prospective study. Scot Med J 39(5): 147-9.

Gilling-Smith C, Toozs-Hobson P, Potts DJ *et al* (1998). Failure to comply with anti-D prophylaxis recommendations in accident and emergency departments. Proceedings of the Consensus Conference on Anti-D Prophylaxis. BJOG 105(18): 24.

Glazebrook B, Akers C, Bielby L *et al* (2020). Quality audit of the guidelines for the use of RhD immunoglobulin in obstetrics: Are we getting it right? ANZJOG 60(4): 504-08.

Hamel C, Esmaeilisaraji L, Thuku M *et al* (2020). Antenatal and postpartum prevention of Rh alloimmunization: A systematic review and GRADE analysis. PLoS ONE 15(9): e0238844.

Harkness M (2015). Anti-D: getting it right. RCM Midwives 18:22.

Harkness M, Freer Y & Warner P (2016). Midwives' experience of offering anti-D immunoglobulin to women: The importance of choice. BJM 24(7): 500-05.

Harmon P (1987). Rhogam at 28 weeks. Midwifery Today 4: 24-25.

Hensleigh PA (1983). Preventing rhesus isoimmunization: antepartum Rh immune globulin prophylaxis *versus* a sensitive test for risk identification. AJOG 146: 749-55.

Hoffbrand AV, Lewis SM & Tuddenham EGD (1999). Postgraduate Haematology. 4th ed. Butterworth Heinemann.

Howard HL, Martlew VJ, McFadyn IR *et al* (1997a). Preventing rhesus D haemolytic disease of the newborn by giving anti-D immunoglobulin: are the guidelines being adequately followed? BJOG 194: 37-41.

Howard HL, Martlew VJ, McFadyn IR *et al* (1997b). Current use of anti-D immunoglobulin in preventing rhesus hemolytic disease. CROG 9(3): 181-88.

Huchet J, Dallemagne S, Huchet C *et al* (1987). The antepartum use of anti-D immunoglobulin in rhesus negative women. Parallel evaluation of fetal blood cells passing through the placenta. The results of a multicentre trial carried out in the region of Paris. JGOBR(Paris) 16: 101-11.

Huggon AM & Watson DP (1993). Use of anti-D in an accident and emergency department. Arch Emergency Medicine 10(4), 306-09.

Hughes RG, Craig JL, Murphy WG *et al* (1994). Causes and clinical consequences of rhesus (D) haemolytic disease of the newborn: a study of a Scottish population, 1985-1990. BJOG 101(4): 297-300.

Inch S (1982). Birthrights. A Parents' Guide to Modern Childbirth. London: Hutchinson.

Jacobs W (1956). The use of bioflavinoid compounds in the prevention or reduction in severity of erythroblastosis fetalis. Surge Obstet. Gynecol. August: 233-36.

Jacobs W (1960). Further experience with bioflavinoid compounds in Rh immunized women. Surge Obstet. Gynecol. January: 33-34.

Jacobs W (1965). Citrus bioflavinoid compounds in Rh-immunized gravidas: results of a ten year study. AJOG 25(5): 648-49.

James D (1998). Anti-D prophylaxis in 1997: The Edinburgh Consensus Statement. Arch Dis Childhood: F&N Ed 78(3): F161-65.

Jensen MPS, Damkjær MB, Clausen FB et al (2019). Targeted Rhesus immunoglobulin for RhD-negative women undergoing an induced abortion: A clinical pilot study. AOGS 98(9): 1164-71.

Juul LA, Hartwig TS, Ambye L et al (2020). Non-invasive prenatal testing and maternal obesity - A review. AOGS 99(6): 744-50.

Karanth L, Jaafar SH, Kanagasabai S et al (2013). Anti-D administration after spontaneous miscarriage for preventing Rhesus alloimmunisation. Cochrane Database Syst Rev. 28:(3):CD009617. doi: 10.1002/14651858.CD009617.pub2. PMID: 23543581.

Katz J (1969). Transplacental passage of fetal red cells in abortion; increased incidence after curettage and effect of oxytocic drugs. BMJ 214(4): 84-86.

Katz LM (2020). Is SARS-CoV-2 transfusion transmitted? Transfusion 60(6): 1111-14.

Keith L & Bozorgi N (1977). Small dose Anti-Rh therapy after first trimester abortion. IJGO 15: 235-37.

Kenny-Walsh W (1999). Clinical outcomes after hepatitis C infection from contaminated Anti-D Immune Globulin. NEJM 340: 1228-33.

Kirchebner, C., Solder, E. & Schonitzer, D. (1994). Prevention of rhesus incompatibility and viral safety (in German). Infusionsther Transfusionmed 24(4): 281.

Kirkham M (2018). Standardisation of Care: a contradiction in terms. Midwifery Matters 157: 4-7.

Kumar S & Regan F (2005). Management of pregnancies with RhD alloimmunisation. BMJ 28330(7502): 1255-58.

Lachman E, Hingley SM, Bates G *et al* (1977). Detection and measurement of fetomaternal haemorrhage; serum alpha-protein and Kleihauer technique. BMJ 240(1): 1377-79.

Lee D & Rawlinson VI (1995). Multicentre trial of antepartum low-dose anti-D immunoglobulin. Trans Med 5: 15-19.

Levine P & Stetson R (1939). An unusual case of intra-group agglutination JAMA 113(2): 126-27.

Levine P, Katzin EM & Burnham L (1941). Isoimmunisation in pregnancy. Its possible bearing on the etiology of erythroblastosis fetalis. JAMA 116: 825-27.

Liumbruno GM, D'Alessandro A, Rea F *et al* (2010). The role of antenatal immunoprophylaxis in the prevention of maternal-foetal anti-Rh(D) alloimmunisation. Blood Transfusion 8(1): 8-16.

Maayan-Metzger A, Schwartz T, Sulkes J *et al* (2001). Maternal anti-D prophylaxis during pregnancy does not cause neonatal haemolysis. Arch Dis Childhood: F&N Ed 84: F60–F62.

Maayan-Metzger A, Leibovitch L, Schushan-Eisen I *et al* (2014). Maternal anti-D prophylaxis during pregnancy and risk of hemolysis among preterm infants J Perinatology 34: 906-08.

Malviya AN, Tripathy S, Chaudhary K *et al* (1989). The anti-D vaccine episode; lessons for everyone in the HIV field. CARC Calling 2: 12.

Manzanares S, Entrala C, Sanchez-Gila M *et al* (2014). Noninvasive Fetal RhD Status Determination in Early Pregnancy. Fetal Diagnosis and Therapy 35(1): 7-12.

Mayne S, Parker JH, Dodds SD *et al* (1997). Rate of RhD sensitisation before and after implementation of a community based antenatal prophylaxis programme. BMJ 315: 1588.

McBain RD, Crowther CA & Middleton P (2015). Anti-D administration in pregnancy for preventing Rhesus alloimmunisation. Cochrane Database of Systematic Reviews 2015, Issue 9. Art. No.: CD000020. DOI: 10.1002/14651858.CD000020.pub3

McSweeney E, Kirkham J, Vinall P *et al* (1998). An audit of anti-D sensitisation in Yorkshire. BJOG 105: 1091-94.

Meisel H, Reip A & Faltus B. (1995). Transmission of hepatitis C virus to children and husbands by women infected with contaminated anti-D immunoglobulin. Lancet 345(8589): 1209-11.

Miles JH & Kaback MD (1979). Rh immune globulin after genetic amniocentesis. Clin Gen Res 27: I03A.

Miller S, Abalos E, Chamillard M *et al* (2016). Beyond too little, too late and too much, too soon: a pathway towards evidence-based, respectful maternity care. The Lancet 388(10056): 2176-92.

Moise KJ (2002). Management of rhesus alloimmunization in pregnancy. Obstetrics & Gynecology 100(3): 600-11.

Mollison PL, Barron SL, Bowley CC *et al* (1974). Controlled trial of various anti-D dosages in suppression of Rh sensitisation following pregnancy: report to the MRC by the Working Party on the use of anti-D immunoglobulin for the prevention of isoimmunization of Rh-negative women during pregnancy. BMJ 2: 75-80.

Morrison J (2000). Audit of anti-D immunoglobulin administration to pregnant Rhesus D negative women following sensitising events. JOG 20(4): 371-73.

Neovius M, Tiblad E, Westgren M *et al* (2016). Cost-effectiveness of first trimester non-invasive fetal RHD screening for targeted antenatal anti-D prophylaxis in RhD-negative pregnant women: a model-based analysis. BJOG 123(8):1337-46.

NHS (2021). Newborn Jaundice.
www.nhs.uk/conditions/jaundice-newborn/

NICE (2016). High-throughput non-invasive prenatal testing for fetal RHD genotype. Diagnostics guidance [DG25] London: NICE.
www.nice.org.uk/guidance/dg25/chapter/4-Evidence

Plested M & Kirkham M (2016). Risk and fear in the lived experience of birth without a midwife. Midwifery 38: 29-34.

Prusova K, Tyler A, Churcher L & Lokugamage AU (2014). Royal College of Obstetricians and Gynaecologists guidelines: How evidence-based are they? JOG 34(8): 706-11.

Reilly M & Lawlor E (1999). A likelihood-based method of identifying contaminated lots of blood product. Int J Epid 28(4): 787-92.

Qureshi H, Massey E, Kirwan D *et al* (2014). BCSH guideline for the use of anti-D immunoglobulin for the prevention of haemolytic disease of the fetus and newborn. Transfusion Medicine 24(1): 8-20.

RANZCOG (2019). Guidelines for the use of Rho(D) immune-globulin in obstetrics. Melbourne: RANZCOG.

Robson SC, Lee D & Urbaniak S (1998). Anti-D immuneglobulin in RhD prophylaxis. BJOG 105: 129-34.

Romm AV (1999). Rho(D) immune globulin: pros, cons, indications and alternatives. Birth Gazette 15(2): 18-21.

Rowley M, Davies T, Grant-Casey J *et al* (2013). National Comparative Audit of Blood Transfusion. 2013 Audit of Anti-D Immuno-globulin Prophylaxis. RCP and NHS Blood & Transport.

Royal College of Midwives (1999). Anti-D update. RCM Midwives Journal November 1999 mid-month supplement.

Runkel B, Bein G, Sieben W *et al* (2020). Targeted antenatal anti-D prophylaxis for RhD-negative pregnant women: a systematic review. BMC Pregnancy and Childbirth 20(83).

Rutkowski K & Nasser SM (2014). Management of hypersensitivity reactions to anti-D immunoglobulin preparations. Allergy 69(11): 1560-63.

Saha A. (1998). Women should be counselled about source of anti-D immunoglobulin (letter). BMJ 316: 1164.

Schochow & Steger (2020). Medical care or clinical research on humans? Contaminated anti-D immunoglobulin in the GDR and its consequences. (Medizinische Versorgung oder Klinische Forschung am Menschen? Die kontaminierte Anti-D-Immunprophylaxe in der DDR und ihre Folgen). Z Gastroenterol 58(02): 127-32.

Schlensker KH & Kruger AA (1996). Results of postpartum prophylaxis 1967-1990 (in German). G Frauenheilkd 56(9): 494-500.

Smits-Wintjens VEHJ & Lopriore FJWE (2008). Rhesus haemolytic disease of the newborn: Postnatal management, associated morbidity and long-term outcome. Seminars in Fetal and Neonatal Medicine 13(4): 265-71.

Sperling JD, Dahlke JD, Sutton D *et al* (2018). Prevention of RhD Alloimmunization: A Comparison of Four National Guidelines. American Journal of Perinatology 35(02): 110-19.

Standing Medical Advisory Committee (1976). Haemolytic Disease of the Newborn. London: Department of Health and Social Security.

Standing Medical Advisory Committee (1976 - addendum 1981). Memorandum on Haemolytic Disease of the Newborn. London: Department of Health and Social Security.

Stenchever MA, Davies IJ, Weisman R *et al* (1970). Rho(D) immune-globulin: a double blind clinical trial. AJOG 106(2), 316-17.

Stine LE, Phelan JP, Do RW *et al* (1985). Update on external version performed at term. OG 65: 642-46.

Tabsh KMA, Lebherz TB & Crandall BF (1984). Risks of prophylactic anti-D immunoglobulin after second-trimester amniocentesis. AJOG 149(2): 225-26.

Teitelbaum L, Metcalfe A. Clarke G *et al* (2015). Costs and benefits of non-invasive fetal RhD determination. Ultrasound in Obstetrics and Gynecology 45(1): 84-88.

Thornton JG, Page C, Foote G *et al* (1989). Efficacy and long term effects of antenatal prophylaxis with anti-D immunoglobulin. BMJ 298: 1671.

Tneh SY, Baidya S, Daly J (2020). Clinical practices and outcomes of RhD immunoglobulin prophylaxis following large-volume fetomaternal haemorrhage in Queensland, Australia. ANZJOG ajo.13226.

Tovey LAD (1986). Haemolytic disease of the newborn: the changing scene. BJOG 93(9): 960-66.

Tovey LAD, Townley A, Stevenson BJ *et al* (1983). The Yorkshire antenatal anti-D immunoglobulin trial in primigravidae. Lancet 1983(ii): 244-46.

Tyndall C, Cuzzilla R & Kane SC (2020). The rhesus incompatible pregnancy and its consequences for affected fetuses and neonates. Transfusion and Apheresis Science 59(5): 102948.

Uldbjerg N (2017). No-call non-invasive prenatal testing gives important information. BJOG 125(7): 856.

Urbaniak S (1998). Proceedings of the Consensus Conference on Anti-D prophylaxis. JOG 105(18): 24.

Vege S & Westhoff CM (2019). Rh and RhAG Blood Group Systems. In: Shaz BH, Hillyer CD & Reyes Gil M (Eds) (2019). Transfusion Medicine and Hemostasis (Third Edition). Elsevier. 149-55.

Visscher RD & Visscher HC (1972). Do Rh-negative women with an early spontaneous abortion need Rh immuno prophylaxis? AJOG 113: 158-65.

Visser GHA, Di Renzo GC, Spitalnik SL *et al* (2019). The continuing burden of Rh disease 50 years after the introduction of anti-Rh(D) immunoglobin prophylaxis: call to action. AJOG 221(3): 227.e1-e4.

Vivanti A, Benachi A, Huchet F-X *et al* (2016). Diagnostic accuracy of fetal rhesus D genotyping using cell-free fetal DNA during the first trimester of pregnancy. AJOG 215(5): 606.e1–606.e5.

Vos GH (1967). The effect of external version on antenatal immunization by the Rh factor. Vox Sang 12: 390-96.

Wagner FF, Gassner C, Müller DS (1999). Molecular basis of weak D phenotypes. Blood 93: 385-93.

White CA, Visscher RD, Visscher HC *et al* (1970). Rho(D) immune prophylaxis: a double blind co-operative study. OG 36(3): 341-46.

White CA, Stedman CM, Frank S *et al* (1983). Anti-D antibodies in D- and Du-positive women: A cause of hemolytic disease of the newborn. AJOG 145(8): 1069-73.

White SW, Cheng JC, Penova-Veselinovic B *et al* (2019). Single dose *v* two-dose antenatal anti-D prophylaxis: a randomised controlled trial. MJA 211(6): 261-65.

Wickham S (2001). Anti-D in Midwifery: panacea or paradox? Oxford: Books for Midwives Press.

Wickham S (2005). Anti-D: helping women make informed choices. BJM 13(4): 225-28.

Wickham S (2017). Vitamin K and the Newborn. Avebury: Birthmoon Creations.

Wickham S (2018a). What's Right For Me? Making decisions in pregnancy and childbirth. Avebury: Birthmoon Creations.

Wickham, S (2018b). Inducing Labour: making informed decisions. Avebury: Birthmoon Creations.

Wickham S (2019). Group B Strep Explained. Avebury: Birthmoon Creations.

World Health Organization (1971). Prevention of Rh Sensitization. Technical Reports No 468. Geneva: World Health Organization.

Yap PL (1997). Viral transmission by blood products: a perspective of events covered by the recent tribunal of enquiry into the Irish Blood Transfusion Board. Irish Med J 90(3): 84, 86, 88.

Yazer MH & Triulzi DJ (2007). Detection of anti-D in D- recipients transfused with D+ red blood cells. Transfusion 47: 2197-2201.

Zhu YJ, Zheng YR, Li L *et al* (2014). Diagnostic accuracy of non-invasive fetal RhD genotyping using cell-free fetal DNA: a meta analysis. J M-FNM 27(18): 1839-44.

Zipursky A & Israels LG (1967). The pathogenesis and prevention of Rh immunization. CMAJ 97(21): 1245057.

Zwiers C, Koelewijn JM, Vermij L *et al* (2018). ABO incompatibility and RhIG immunoprophylaxis protect against non-D alloimmunization by pregnancy. Transfusion 58: 1611-17.

Also by Sara Wickham

In Your Own Time: how western medicine controls the start of labour and why this needs to stop

Pregnant women and maternity services are facing an induction epidemic. In this timely book, Dr Sara Wickham demystifies the evidence and highlights the significant discrepancies between guidelines and what we really know about the benefits of supporting women to birth spontaneously. In Your Own Time details how we got to this state and looks at the evidence relating to due dates, 'post-term', older and larger women, suspected big babies, maternal race and more.

Plus Size Pregnancy: what the evidence really says about higher BMI and birth

Sara looks at the evidence relating to higher BMI and birth, unpacking the myths, explaining the evidence, and helping you understand your options. Reviewers describe it as, "a game changer," "truly filled with so much useful knowledge," and said, "I wish I got this book way sooner, the anxiety it would've saved."

Inducing Labour: making informed decisions

Sara's bestselling book explains the process of induction of labour and shares information from research studies, debates and women's, midwives' and doctors' experiences to help women and families get informed and decide what is right for them.

Group B Strep Explained

Explains everything that parents and birth workers need to know about Group B Strep; a common and usually harmless bacteria which can occasionally cause problems for babies. Sara discusses screening, preventative measures, alternatives and wider issues.

Also by Sara Wickham

Vitamin K and the Newborn

Find out everything you need to know about vitamin K; why it's offered to newborn babies, why are there different viewpoints on it and what do parents need to know in order to make the decision that is right for them and their baby?

What's Right For Me? Making decisions in pregnancy and childbirth

The decisions that we make about our childbirth journeys can shape our experiences, health and lives, and those of our families. A guide to the different approaches that exist; offering information, tips and tools to help you make the decisions that are right for you.

Birthing Your Placenta (with Nadine Edwards)

A popular book which helps parents, professionals and others to understand the process and the evidence relating to the birth of the placenta. No matter what kind of birth you are hoping for, this book will help you understand the issues and options.

101 tips for planning, writing and surviving your dissertation

These 101 tips are useful for students at any stage of their academic career. Written in an accessible, friendly style and seasoned with first-hand advice, this book combines sound, practical tips from an experienced academic with reminders of the value of creativity, chocolate and naps in your work.

Made in the USA
Monee, IL
11 November 2024

69873966R00098